The Brain: A Very Short Introduction

Very Short Introductions available now:

Michael O'Shea

THE BRAIN

A Very Short Introduction

OXFORD
UNIVERSITY PRESS

OXFORD
UNIVERSITY PRESS

Great Clarendon Street, Oxford OX2 6DP

Oxford University Press is a department of the University of Oxford.
It furthers the University's objective of excellence in research, scholarship,
and education by publishing worldwide in

Oxford New York

Auckland Cape Town Dar es Salaam Hong Kong Karachi
Kuala Lumpur Madrid Melbourne Mexico City Nairobi
New Delhi Shanghai Taipei Toronto

With offices in

Argentina Austria Brazil Chile Czech Republic France Greece
Guatemala Hungary Italy Japan Poland Portugal Singapore
South Korea Switzerland Thailand Turkey Ukraine Vietnam

Oxford is a registered trade mark of Oxford University Press
in the UK and in certain other countries

Published in the United States
by Oxford University Press Inc., New York

© Michael O'Shea 2005

The moral rights of the author have been asserted
Database right Oxford University Press (maker)

First published as a Very Short Introduction 2005

All rights reserved. No part of this publication may be reproduced,
stored in a retrieval system, or transmitted, in any form or by any means,
without the prior permission in writing of Oxford University Press,
or as expressly permitted by law, or under terms agreed with the appropriate
reprographics rights organizations. Enquiries concerning reproduction
outside the scope of the above should be sent to the Rights Department,
Oxford University Press, at the address above

You must not circulate this book in any other binding or cover
and you must impose this same condition on any acquirer

British Library Cataloguing in Publication Data
Data available

Library of Congress Cataloging in Publication Data
Data available

ISBN 978–0–19–285392–9

13 15 17 19 20 18 16 14

Typeset by RefineCatch Ltd, Bungay, Suffolk
Printed in Great Britain by
Ashford Colour Press Ltd, Gosport, Hants

To my children Annie and Jack. And to my daughter Linda who died because not enough was known about what to do when stuff goes seriously wrong in the brain. I hope that some day we shall know enough.

Contents

Acknowledgements

I thank Annalie Clark for her intelligent advice, especially on improving the clarity of the difficult bits. Dr Liz Somerville for her expert tutorial on the fossilized antecedents of the human cranium. Also Jenny for her encouragement.

List of illustrations

Chapter 1
Thinking about the brain

Think for a few moments about a very special machine, your brain –
an organ of just 1.2 kg, containing one hundred billion nerve cells,
none of which alone has any idea who or what you are. In fact the
very idea that a cell can have an idea seems silly. A single cell after
all is far too simple an entity. However, conscious awareness of one's
self comes from just that: nerve cells communicating with one
another by a hundred trillion interconnections. When you think
about it this is a deeply puzzling fact of life. It may not be entirely
unreasonable therefore to suppose that such a machine must be
endowed with miraculous properties. But while the world is full of
mystery, science has no place for miracles and the 21st century's
most challenging scientific problem is nothing short of explaining
how the brain works in purely material terms.

Thinking about your brain is itself something of a conundrum
because you can only think about your brain *with* your brain.
You'll appreciate the curious circularity of this riddle if you
consider the consequence of concluding, as you might, that your
brain is the most exquisitely complex and extraordinary machine
in the known universe. Clearly this is, and may be nothing more
than, the opinion of your brain about *itself*: the brain's way of
thinking about the brain. So it seems we are caught in the logical
paradox of a self-referencing, and in this case also a self-obsessed,
system. Perhaps the only reliable conclusion from this thought

experiment is that the brain is about as conceited as it is possible to be!

Notwithstanding the brain's well-developed personal vanity, we must grant that it provides you with some very distinctive abilities. It operates in the background of your every action, sensation, and thought. It allows you to reflect vividly on the past, to make informed judgements about the present, and to plan rational courses of action into the future. It endows you with the seemingly effortless ability to form pictures in your mind, to perceive music in noise, to dream, to dance, to fall in love, cry, and laugh. Perhaps most remarkable of all however is the brain's ability to generate conscious awareness, which convinces you that you are *free to choose* what you will do next.

We have no idea how consciousness arises from a physical machine and in trying to understand how the brain does that we may well be up against the most awkward of scientific challenges. That is not to say that the problem cannot in principle be solved, just that the brain is a finite machine and presumably has a finite capacity for understanding. But what are the limits of its intellectual capacity and, at that limit, might we still be asking unanswerable questions about the brain? Neuroscientists accept that they are faced with an awesome challenge. The accelerating pace of discovery in neuroscience however shows that we are a long way from any theoretical upper limit on our capacity for understanding that might exist. So rather than despairing of the limitations of the human intellect, we should be optimistic in our striving for a complete physical understanding of the brain and of its most puzzling of properties – consciousness and the sensation of free will.

Although we have barely started this short book we have already made a fundamental conceptual error in the way we have referred to 'the brain'. The brain is not an independent agent, residing in splendid and lofty superiority in our skulls. Rather it is part of an extended system reaching out to permeate, influence, and be influenced by, every corner and extremity of your body. As the spinal cord, your brain extends the length of the backbone, periodically sprouting nerves that convey information to and from every part of you. Practically nothing is out of its reach. Every breath you take, every beat of your heart, your every emotion, every movement, including involuntary ones such as the bristling of the hairs on the back of your neck and the movement of food through your guts – all of these are controlled directly or indirectly by the action of the nervous system, of which the brain is the ultimate part.

From this perspective the brain is not simply a centre for issuing instructions, it is itself bombarded by a constant barrage of information flowing in from our bodies and the outside world. Specialized cells called sensory receptor neurons feed information via sensory nerves into the nervous system, providing the brain with real-time data on both the internal state of the body and about the outside world. Furthermore, information flowing into and out of the brain is carried not only by nerve cells. About 20 per cent of the volume of the brain is occupied by blood vessels, which supply the oxygen and glucose for the brain's exceptionally high energy demand. The blood supply provides an alternative communication channel between the brain and the body and between the body and brain. Endocrine glands throughout the body release hormones into the blood stream. These hormones inform the brain about the state of bodily functions, whilst the brain deposits hormonal instructions into its blood supply for distribution globally to the rest of the body. So when we say the brain does x or y, the word 'brain' is a shorthand for all of the interdependent interactive processes of a complex dynamical system consisting of the brain, the body, and the outside world.

The human brain is a highly evolved and stupendously complex 'machine' that is often compared to the most complex of man-made machines, digital computers. But brains and computers differ fundamentally. The brain is an evolved biological entity made from materials such as small organic molecules, proteins, lipids, and carbohydrates, a few trace elements, and quite a lot of salty water. A modern computer is built with electronic components and switches made from silicon, metal, and plastic. Does it *matter* what a machine is made of? For computers the answer is no – computer operations are 'medium independent'. That is to say, any computation can in principle be performed in any medium, using components made from any suitable material. Thus cogs and levers, hydraulics or optical devices for that matter could replace the electronics of a modern computer, without affecting (except in terms of speed and convenience) the machine's ability to compute. It seems extraordinarily unlikely either that the brain is simply performing computational algorithms or that thinking could equally well be achieved with cogs and levers as with nerve cells. So perhaps we cannot expect computers to perform like brains unless we find a way to build them in a biological medium (see Chapter 7).

From marks to meaning

To gain an insight into questions about the brain that must be answered, and to set the stage for later chapters, I will now briefly examine the activity of the brain in the context of a familiar act of everyday life. Let us consider the behaviour in which you are currently engaged – namely, reading these words. What exactly is your brain is doing right now? What kind of behaviour is reading and what must the brain do in order to achieve it?

Obviously the brain must first learn how to read and equally obviously reading is a means of learning and engages our imagination. Reading also demands concentration and attention. Therefore as you read these words your brain must direct your attention away from the many potential distractions that are constantly in the background, all around you. You need not worry however because, without bothering your conscious awareness, your brain is keeping a watchful 'eye' on external events. It can at any moment redirect your attention away from this page and towards something more important. Your attention can also be distracted by events internal to the brain, the various thoughts that constantly pass through it and compete for your consciousness.

Reading, when reduced to the rather prosaic level of motor actions, depends on the brain's ability to orchestrate a series of eye movements. Now, as you read these words, your brain is commanding your eyes to make small but very rapid (about 500° per second) left-to-right movements called saccades (right-to-left or up-and-down for some other written languages). You are not consciously aware of it, but these rapid movements are frequently interrupted by brief periods when the eyes are fixed in position. Watch someone reading and you will see exactly what I mean. You'll notice that the eyes do not sweep smoothly along the line of text, rather they dart from one fixation to another. It is only during the fixations, when the eyes dwell for about a fifth of a second, that the brain is able to examine the text in detail. Reading is not possible during the darting saccadic movements because the eyes are moving too quickly across the page. You are not aware of the blur and confusion during a saccade because fortunately there is a brain mechanism that suppresses vision and protects you from visual overload.

Reading is only possible between saccades, not only because the eyes are then stationary but also because gaze is centred on the retina's fovea. The fovea is the only part of the retina specialized for high acuity vision (see Chapter 5), but it scrutinizes a very small area of our visual world. As a literal rule of thumb, foveal vision is restricted approximately to the area of your vision covered by your thumbnail held at arm's length. It is a small window of clear vision within which you are able to decipher just 7 or 8 letters of normal print size at a time. The task for the brain is to generate a precise series of motor commands to the eye muscles which ensure that at the end of each saccade your high acuity vision is fixed on that part of the text you need to see most clearly *next*. As your eyes approach the end of a line, the brain generates a carriage return. Of course the return saccade must be to the left, of the correct magnitude and associated with a slight downward shift in gaze in order to bring the first word on the next line onto the fovea.

I have considered only the simple case of the brain directing eye movements alone, as if nothing else affects gaze direction. But of course the relative positions of the eye and page are affected continuously by head, body, and book motion. Thus the brain must continually monitor and anticipate factors affecting the future position of your eyes relative to the text. The fact that you can effortlessly read on a moving train while eating a sandwich is evidence that your brain can solve this problem quite easily. Importantly, it is done automatically and on an unconscious level without you having to think through every step. If you had to consciously think about the mechanical process of reading, you would be illiterate!

Our lack of conscious awareness of underlying brain processes can also be illustrated by reflecting on the subjective experience that the comprehension of written material represents. While reading we are not conscious of the fragmented nature of comprehension imposed by underlying *move—stop—move—stop* activity of the eyes I've just described or by the fact that only 7 or 8 letters can be deciphered at each stop. On the contrary, our strong subjective impression is that comprehension of the text flows uninterrupted and moreover that we can read several words or even whole sentences 'at a glance'. That this is not the case can be illustrated by reading a sentence containing a word that has more than one meaning and pronunciation. For example, the word *tear* has two very different meanings and pronunciations in English – tear the noun of crying and tear the verb of ripping apart. Clearly such word ambiguity complicates the brain's task of providing you with an uninterrupted comprehension. If for instance the word *tear* occurred at the beginning of a sentence its meaning might remain ambiguous until the subject of the sentence appears later. Because you cannot read the whole sentence at a glance your brain may be left with no option but to choose one of the alternative meanings (or sounds, if you are reading aloud) of a word and hope for the best.

While we cannot read whole sentences at a glance, the brain does recognize each word as a whole. What is quite surprising however is that the order of the letters is not particularly important (good news for poor spellers). That is why you will be able to read the following passage without consciously having to decode it.

I cdnuolt blveiee taht I cluod aulaclty uesdnatnrd waht I was rdgnieg. It deosn't mttaer in waht oredr the ltteers in a wrod aer, the olny iprmoatnt tihng is taht eth frist dan lsat ltteer be in the rghit pclae. The rset cna be a taotl mses and yuo can still raed it wouthit a porbelm. Tihs is bcuseae the huamn mnid deos not raed ervey lteter by istlef, but the wrod as a wlohe. Amzanig huh?

We will now consider how and in what form textual information at the gaze point enters the brain. Light-sensitive cells called photoreceptors capture light focused as two slightly different images on the left and right retinae. The photoreceptors undertake a fundamental and remarkable transformation of energy, a transformation that must occur for all of our senses. This process is known as *sensory transduction* and always involves converting the energy in the sensory stimulus, in this case light energy, into an electrical signal. This is because the nervous system cannot use light or sound or touch or smell directly as a currency of information transmission. In the brain electricity is the critically important currency of information flow.

The brain interprets or decodes electrical signals according to their address and destination. We *see* an electrical signal coming from the eyes, *hear* electrical signals from the ears, and *feel* the electrical signals coming from touch sensitive cells in the skin. You can demonstrate the importance of signal origin by pressing very gently with your little finger into the corner of your closed right eye, next to your nose. The touch pressure will locally distort the retina and produce an electrical signal that will be transmitted to the brain. Your brain will 'see' a small spot of light in the visual field caused by touch. Notice that the light appears to be coming from the peripheral visual field somewhere off to the right; a moment's thought should tell you why this is so.

The photoreceptor cells of the retina are not connected directly to the brain. They communicate with a network of retinal neurons through a mechanism that couples the fluctuating electrical signal in the photoreceptor to the release of a variety of chemicals known as neurotransmitters. In their turn, neurotransmitters convey signals from one neuron to another by generating or suppressing electrical signals in neighbouring neurons that are specifically sensitive to particular neurotransmitters. This transformation of an electrical into a chemical signal occurs mostly at specialized sites called chemical synapses. Electrical signals can also pass directly between neurons at sites known as electrical synapses. Thus, through a combination of direct electrical transmission between neurons and the release of chemical messengers, information about the visual image captured by the eyes is processed in the retina before being conveyed by the optic nerve to the brain.

There are about one million output neurons in the retina, known as retinal ganglion cells, and each one extends a long, slender fibre or axon in the optic nerve. Axons are specialized for the high-speed (up to 120m/second), long-distance, and faithful transmission of brief electrical impulses. Impulses travelling along the axons of the retinal ganglion cells in the optic nerve reach the first neurons in the brain about 35 thousandths of a second after the capture of photons by the photoreceptors. In the brain, the axons of the retinal ganglion cells terminate and form synapses with a variety of other neurons which in turn interconnect with many others, a process which results finally in the conscious awareness of a vivid picture in your mind of what your eyes are looking at. Somehow this astonishing electrochemical process that involves no conscious effort whatsoever produces meaningful pictures in your mind – close your eyes and the picture goes away, open them and it appears to you apparently instantaneously and effortlessly. Truly amazing!

Reading does not come naturally; it is a difficult skill that must be acquired painfully. Once learnt however it is rarely, if ever, forgotten – thankfully. So we do not have to worry about forgetting how to read because the skill is robustly established in our long-term memory banks. Although the enabling skill of reading is retained in permanent memory, an entirely different type of memory is required during the active process of reading itself. While reading, we must retain a short-term 'working memory' for what has just been read. Some of the information acquired while reading may be committed to long-term memory but much is remembered for just long enough to enable you to understand the text. Memories must somehow be represented *physically* in the brain. Brain chemistry and structure is altered by experience and the stability of these physicochemical changes presumably corresponds to the retention duration of memory. So what exactly is a memory? What kind of physical trace is left in the brain after we have learnt some new skill or fact? What is forgetting and why are some memories quickly forgotten and others never? These are questions to which I shall return later.

Finally we must consider one of the most elusive of problems. While accepting that everything that the brain does depends on lawful processes occurring within and between the brain's cells, how can we explain how 'meanings' arise in our minds while reading words? How do marks on paper become images in the mind, how do they make you think? How can any of this be explained completely by the responses of individual brain cells and interactions between them? Consider for example what happens when I recognize the word banana. I instantly call up an image of a yellow, curved object about 20 cm in length, 4 cm in girth, that is edible and incidentally delicious. We might propose that there is a single neuron in my brain that responds when I read 'banana' and triggers all of the remembered associated thoughts. Maybe this is the same neuron that responds when I see a real banana.

According to this logic, a different neuron fires when I look at an apple and another recognizes my grandmother. While it is true that neurons can respond rather specifically to particular stimuli, most neuroscientists believe that there can be no one-to-one correspondence between the response of an individual neuron and a perception. Surely a separate neuron cannot detect and represent every object and percept? After all, in order to know that that object is a banana, information about shape, size, texture, and colour must somehow be bound together with stored knowledge about fruit, my appetite, and so on. These processes are associated with different networks of neurons in different parts of the brain and there is no known way they could all converge on a single neuron which when activated could trigger 'aha, a banana for lunch'. Another way to think about the relationship between the activities of neurons and a perception is to consider how assemblies of nerve cells in different parts of the brain cooperate with one another in parallel. Having said that, we are far from understanding how objects, meanings, and perceptions are encoded in the brain by the activities of neurons. This is one of the most intriguing of problems in neuroscience. While the notion that there is a separate nerve cell in the brain for each object, meaning, and perception (parodied by the term 'Grandmother cell') has been roundly rejected, there is a lasting appeal in this simple idea. Indeed provocative research published at the time of writing this sheds a fresh perspective on the way objects are represented in the brain. It suggests that the idea there may be a neuron in your brain that only recognizes your grandmother deserves some serious reconsideration – I shall return to this matter later.

In the following chapters of this book I shall examine in more detail the questions and issues considered in this introduction. Starting with a historical perspective on the development of modern brain science I go on to describe electrical and chemical signalling mechanisms that underlie all mental functions, how the nervous systems evolved, how the brain responds to sensations and perceptions, the formation of memories and what can be done when the brain is damaged. The potential for interfacing the brain with computers is discussed, as is the contribution of neuroscience to developments in robotics and artificial nervous systems. Finally, I discuss the future scientific challenges associated with understanding how the brain works as a whole.

Chapter 2
From humours to cells: components of mind

The widespread occurrence of the 'surgical' technique of trepanation, the removal of parts of skull to expose the brain, in early civilizations suggests that ancient cultures recognized the brain as a critical organ. This is not to suggest that a link between the brain and the mind has its roots in prehistory. In fact the long history of neuroscience prior to the scientific period suggests that it is not at all self-evident that mental functions must necessarily be attributed to the brain. The Egyptians for instance clearly did not hold the brain in particularly high esteem since in the process of mummification it was scooped out and discarded (a practice that stopped around the end of the 2nd century AD). To the ancient Egyptians, it was the heart that was credited with intelligence and thought – probably for this reason it was carefully preserved when mummifying the deceased.

Although Hippocrates (460–370 BC) is usually accredited with being the first in the West to argue that the brain is the most important organ for sensation, thought, emotion, and cognition, he was not the first Greek to consider the question of physical embodiment of mind. Prior to the Hippocratic revolution, Pythagoras (582–500 BC) believed that matter and mind are connected somehow and that the mind is attuned to the laws of mathematics. It was probably of little interest to Pythagoras whether mind and matter were connected in the brain or, as the Egyptians and the Greeks prior to 500 BC believed, in the heart.

Alcmaeon of Croton (b. 535 BC), himself a follower of Pythagoras, is among the first to have realized that the brain is the likely centre of the intellect. He is also the first known to have conducted human dissections and in doing so he noticed that the eye is connected to the brain by what we now know is the optic nerve. It was on the basis of his direct observations that Alcmaeon astutely speculated, a century before Hippocrates came to a similar conclusion, that the brain was the centre of mental activity. Hippocrates went further than this however and elaborated a theory of four humours that together were responsible for the temperament. Thus, according to Hippocrates, the four determinants of temperament were black bile (melancholy), yellow bile (irascibility), phlegm (equanimity and sluggishness), and sanguine (passion and cheerfulness). To us the humoral theory seems implausible, puzzling, and arbitrary. It seems to have been inspired, not by the evidence of observation, but by the need to conform with the equally unlikely postulates of contemporary Greek natural law, namely that there are four elements: earth, air, water, and fire.

The influence of Hippocrates was to be profound and remarkably long lasting. Some 400 years after Hippocrates died, Claudius Galenus of Pergamum (AD 131–201), better known as Galen, became the most influential physician of his time, in part by building his own theory on the humoral conjectures of Hippocrates. Galen was unusually well informed on the internal anatomy of the human body, an intimate understanding of which he gained while he was physician at a school for gladiators. However, although we can be grateful to him for perpetuating the idea that the brain is the seat of the mind, he continued the Hippocratic tradition of disregarding the importance of the solid tissues of the brain for mental functions. Instead Galen associated the presence in the brain of three fluid filled cavities, or ventricles, with the tripartite division of mental faculties – the rational soul – into imagination, reason, and memory. According to Galen, the brain's primary function is to distribute vital fluid from the ventricles through the nerves to the muscles and organs, thereby somehow controlling bodily activity. Precisely how the brain's ventricles were supposed to regulate the three cognitive functions is not explained, unsurprisingly.

Galen's positive contribution to medical knowledge is undeniable, but many of his ideas were seriously flawed. This would not have mattered too much were it not for the fact that, after he died, Galen's authority dominated and therefore hampered medical science and practice for some 400 years. A particularly interesting example of his influence can be seen in the early anatomical drawings of Leonardo da Vinci (1452–1519). In one drawing of the head, the brain is depicted crudely consisting of three simple cavities labelled O, M, and N. Leonardo interpreted the anatomical division in functional terms in a way that would have been immediately recognizable to Galen in the 1st century.

Later Leonardo was to make some of the most important observations on the brain and its ventricles. He can be credited with the first recorded use of solidifying wax injection to make castings to study the internal cavities of the brain and other organs, including the heart. Using this method, Leonardo accurately determined the shape and extent of the brain's cavities, but he clearly continued to place a Galenical interpretation on the fluid-filled structures. For instance the lateral ventricles carry the word *imprensiva* (perceptual) in Leonardo's hand, the third ventricle is labelled *sensus communis*, and the fourth ventricle, *memoria*. Leonardo's use of wax injections represented a scientific advance of enormous potential and importance. Unfortunately, the dominance of Galen's conjectures about the functions of the ventricles diverted his attention from the solid tissue of the brain, the true seat of the mind.

Ideas about brain function and mechanisms continued to be

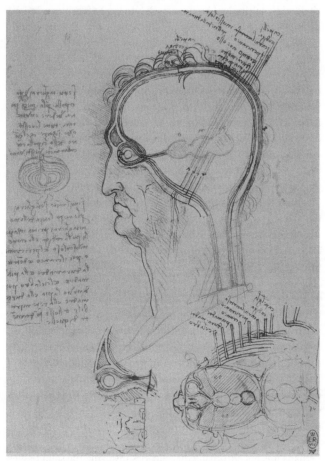

1. Anatomical drawing by Leonardo da Vinci: The human head and its contents according to Leonardo da Vinci. Probably drawn c.1490, it represents an attempt to translate a description of the brain given by medieval philosophers. This drawing shows (wrongly) that the eye is connected by its optic nerve to three simple cavities labelled O, M and N. Leonardo ignores the intricate structure of the solid tissues of the brain. The smaller drawings include a section of an onion (accurate), the eye and orbit and a horizontal section of the head

strongly influenced by theories involving the flow and distillation of vital fluids, spirits, and humours well into the 17th century. Indeed the influence of Hippocrates and Galen can be seen in the hydraulic model of the brain formulated by the most famous 17th-century French philosopher, René Descartes (1596–1650). Descartes however reformulated the humour-based description of the brain's functioning and expressed it in contemporary terms by comparing the brain to the working of intricate machines of his time, such as clocks and moving statues, the movements of which were controlled by hydraulic systems. Importantly he departed from the classical tradition of locating cognitive processes exclusively in the brain's fluid-filled ventricles, but he nonetheless still referred to the flow of spirits through nerves and made no attempt to assign functions to specific brain structures, with the notable exception of the pineal gland. The pineal, because it was a unitary and central structure, was supposed to be the link with the singular soul but was also given executive control, directing the flow of animal spirits through the brain.

In one important respect Descartes was breaking new ground. By comparing the workings of the brain with that of complex hydraulic machines, he was regarding the most technologically advanced artefacts of his day as templates for understanding the brain. This is a tradition that persists today; when we refer to computers and computational operations as models of how the brain acquires, processes, and stores information, for example. So while Descartes was hopelessly wrong in detail, he was adopting a modern style of reasoning.

Perhaps it is not surprising that theories involving the solid tissues of the brain were difficult to conceive – after all, the brain's solid substance has no visible moving parts. By the 17th century, however, the grip of humoral theory was weakening, in part due to the works of a new generation of anatomists who were describing the internal structure of the brain with increasing accuracy. Notably, the Englishman Thomas Willis (1621–75), who coined the term 'neurology', argued that solid cerebral tissue has important functions. He still held that fluid-flow was the key to understanding brain function, but his focus was on the solid cerebral tissues and he showed that nervous function depends on the flow of blood to them. Today's functional brain imaging technique (fMRI) shows that small local increases in blood flow are associated with the activation of nerve cells. That there is in effect a local 'blushing' of the brain when the neurons in that region are active is an observation that Willis might well have expected and enjoyed.

Among the more obvious problems of vital fluid and hydraulic models of nervous system function, and no doubt known to Willis, is that nerves are not hollow conduits. And even if they were, the speed of fluid movement through them could hardly be sufficiently swift for the rapidity with which sensations and motor commands seem to be conveyed by nerves. These and other inconsistencies with fluid models of the nervous system must have worried physicians of the stature of Willis and caused them pause for thought. But Willis remained a fluid theorist and the beginning of the end for the fruitless elaboration of such theories did not come until the discoveries attributed to Luigi Galvani (1737–98). In the late 18th century he discovered the importance of electricity to the operation of the nervous system. As electrical mechanisms were to provide the necessary speed, attention inevitably turned from fluid to electrical models. Ironically, the last gasp of the legacy of Hippocrates and Galen is to be found in the interpretation Galvani himself placed on his own experiments with 'animal electricity'. Having demonstrated that he could control the contractions of a frog muscle by applying electrical currents to the muscle's motor nerve, Galvani claimed to have discovered that animal nerves and muscle contain an electric 'fluid'. A decisive leap of understanding however was achieved when Galvani and his contemporary Alessandro Volta (1745–1827) crucially together linked electricity to the functions of the nervous systems.

What neither Galvani nor Volta could know however is that the externally applied electrical stimuli were activating biological processes causing high-speed electrical impulses to travel along nerves to muscles, resulting in their contraction. It was not until the middle of the 19th century that the ability of nerves and muscles to generate rapidly propagating electrical impulses was confirmed by the German physiologist Du Bois-Reymond (1818–96). This was a major impetus to the study of the physical workings of the brain and set the stage for the modern scientific era, which was launched in a most spectacular way at the dawn of the 20th century by the recognition of the cellular nature of the brain's tiny functional units – the neurons.

The true cellular nature of the brain and of its mental functions was first recognized by the father of modern neuroscience, the Spanish neuroanatomist Santiago Ramon y Cajal (1852–1934). Although his proposition that the brain is a cellular machine may today seem commonplace, in fact it was revolutionary. In the later 19th century, and indeed in the early years of the 20th century, most neuroanatomists believed that the brain was not composed of cells at all – in spite of a universal recognition that all other organs and tissues in our bodies were. What was it about the brain that made it so difficult to see its cellular composition under the microscope? Part of the answer is that brain cells are quite unlike any other cells. The very term 'cell' implies uniformity; simple structures defined by clear boundaries.

In contrast neurons are hugely diverse in morphology. They have exceedingly fine and profusely branched processes ramifying from the cell's body and intermingling among the branches of other neurons. The complexity and diversity of their physical appearance easily exceeds that of all other cell types found in any other part of the body. All of this contributed to a rather confusing picture which anatomists found difficult to reconcile with a simple cellular model of brain structure. When viewed through a microscope the brain appeared to consist of a hopelessly tangled morass (a reticulum), without the distinct cell-defining boundaries that are so evident in

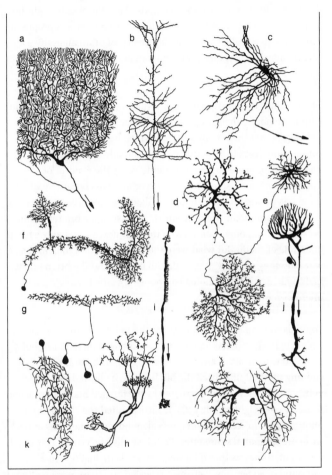

2. A selection of neurons to illustrate diversity: Neurons are more diverse in their appearance than any other type of cell. Their complex branched morphologies are a reflection of their need to communicate with other nearby and more distant neurons. Complexity of shape is no guide to the overall performance of the brain – a neuron in the mammalian brain (top left) is hardly more complicated than a neuron from an insect brain (bottom right)

other tissues. It was therefore not surprising perhaps that cell theory, the idea that tissues are composed of cells, was thought not to apply to the brain and a radical alternative model was proposed. This came to be called the 'reticular theory' of brain anatomy – a surprisingly resilient interpretation that persisted well into the 20th century.

The reticular theory was wrong, but that was not the only problem with it. Scientific theories are allowed to be wrong so long as they are helpful, but the reticular theory, which held that the brain contains no discrete components, was actually obstructive to scientific progress. Progress was hindered by the concept of a machine without discrete functional components because without them it is impossible to formulate a plausible mechanism to explain how the brain might work. Scientists were sure the brain machine *must* have components and, given the complexity of what the brain does, lots of them. But what were they, what did they look like, and what did they do? It was clear that to understand the brain science had to identify the functional components of the brain's microscopic structure.

Towards the end of the 19th century, the Italian anatomist Camillo Golgi (1843–1926) developed a way of highlighting the morphology of very few neurons in any particular region of the brain. It was a staining method that fitted the bill because it allowed individual neurons to be viewed unobstructed by the tangled mass of branched processes of neighbouring cells. It incorporated the chemistry of photographic processing and it revealed individual neurons as dark, silver-impregnated silhouettes. Paradoxically, the crucial feature of Golgi's method was that it hardly ever worked! Just one in a thousand or so neurons were ever revealed and these were scattered more or less randomly throughout the brain tissue. It was precisely because of this uncertain aspect of the method that neurons could for the first time be seen in their entirety disentangled from their neighbours. Immediately it was apparent that there are discrete cells in the brain, but they are astonishing cells – unlike any others.

They differed markedly from one another, in particular with respect to the complex patterns of their numerous branched processes.

Golgi's method was the key to a new set of scientifically testable ideas about how the brain works. The reticular theory was about to be replaced by a far more powerful one called the neuron doctrine, the idea that the brain is composed of discrete cellular components. The neuron doctrine is rightly attributed to Ramon y Cajal who, with the help of Golgi's new staining method, made two profound propositions. The first quite simply is that the neuron is a cell. You might think that this must have been self-evident to anyone who bothered to view a brain treated with Golgi's method. After all, cells in the brain would be clearly visible and thus by the evidence of one's own eyes the reticular theory must be wrong. Somewhat astonishingly, however, in spite of the images provided by his own technique, even Camillo Golgi remained a convinced reticularist.

The second of Cajal's propositions was brilliantly insightful: neurons are structurally *polarized with respect to function*. For the first time, the workings of the brain were explicitly associated with the functions of physical structures at a microscopic level. Cajal concluded that a neuron's function must be concerned with the movement and processing of information in the brain. He could only guess about the form in which information might be encoded or how it might move from place to place. In a stroke of genius, however, he postulated that it would be sensible for the components of function to impose directionality on information flow (or streaming as he called it). So he proposed that information flows in one direction, from an input region to an output region. The neuron's cell body and its shorter processes, known as dendrites, perform input functions. Information then travels along the longest extension from the cell body, known as the axon, to the output region – the terminals of the axon and its branches that contact the input dendrites and cell body of another neuron.

Cajal was fascinated by the differences between the brains of markedly different organisms: human, worms, snails, insects, and so on. He thought comparisons of their brains might be instructive precisely because vast differences exist between the behaviour and intellectual capabilities of different creatures. There is unquestionably an enormous gulf between human and insect intelligence, so it would be reasonable to suppose that a comparison of their brains would expose how structural components reflect intelligence. Surely, the human brain should contain 'high performance' components and the insect brain markedly less sophisticated ones. But the difference between insect and human neurons does not at all betray the gulf between insect and human intelligence. Insect neurons are as complex and display as much diversity as neurons in the human cortex. Cajal himself expressed considerable surprise at this:

> the quality of the psychic machine does not increase with the zoological hierarchy. It is as if we are attempting to equate the qualities of a great wall clock with those of a miniature watch.

Brains of the most advanced insects (honey bees) have about one million neurons, snails about 20,000, and primitive worms (nematodes) about 300. Contrast these numbers with the hundred billion or so that are required for human levels of intelligence. But the individual neurons of simple organisms operate with the very same electrical and chemical signalling machinery found in today's most advanced brains. Like it or not, the astonishing conclusion from comparative studies is that the evolution of our brains, capable of such extraordinary feats, did not require the evolution of 'super neurons'. The basic cellular components of mental functions are pretty much the same in all animals, the humble and the human.

In 1906 Cajal shared the Nobel Prize for Physiology and Medicine with Golgi, 'in recognition of their work on the structure of the nervous system'. This was the first time that the Nobel Prize had been shared between two laureates. The award was controversial because the two disagreed on a crucially important matter – Golgi remained convinced that Cajal was wrong to reject the reticular theory. It was of course Golgi who was wrong and fundamentally so. Other questions over Golgi's interpretations raised serious doubts in the minds of some of the scientists advising the Nobel Council as to the appropriateness of his nomination for the prize. But whatever the merits of the case for a shared prize, 1906 marked the beginning of the modern era in the neurosciences and it was the first of a series of Nobel Prizes to be awarded to neuroscientists over subsequent decades.

Cajal could not have anticipated the extraordinary advances in brain science that were about to be made. His recognition of the neurons as polarized units of information transmission was a defining moment in neuroscience. But at the start of the 20th century many questions about precisely how and in what form neurons signal information in the brain remained unanswered. By the middle of the 20th century, neuroscience had become the fastest growing discipline in the history of scientific endeavour and by the end of that century a more or less complete understanding, in exquisite molecular detail, of how neurons generate electrical and chemical signals would be achieved.

In this very short history of man's discovery of the workings of the brain I cannot avoid reference to the discredited pseudo-science of phrenology, a theory developed by the idiosyncratic Viennese physician Franz Joseph Gall (1758–1828). Gall believed that the brain is the organ of the mind but he went much further and postulated that different distinct faculties of the mind, innate attributes of personality, and intellectual ability, are located in different sites in the brain. Gall reasoned that different individuals will have these innate faculties and that the degree of their development would be reflected in the size of the surface region of the brain that housed that particular faculty. These ideas have a very modern ring to them, but Gall thought that the skull would take the shape of the brain's relief and therefore that the bumps on the surface of the skull could be 'read' as an index of various psychological aptitudes.

The practice of phrenology grew and flourished in Europe and then in America from about 1820, becoming a popular fad in the latter part of the 19th century before effectively dying out early in the 20th century (though in fact the British Phrenological Society was not disbanded until 1967). Its demise in the early 20th century coincided with the rapid accumulation of real evidence for the principle that many discrete mental functions are highly and specifically localized to particular parts of the brain. Much of the evidence came as a consequence of the First World War in the form of the many unfortunate victims of gun-shot and shrapnel lesions to specific regions of the brain that produced reproducible disorders. More recently, functional brain imaging techniques such as fMRI have shown beyond doubt that different cognitive functions are indeed localized to specific parts of the brain. So while the exaggerated claim of phrenologists to be able to read the mind from the bumps on the head was refuted, their premise was vindicated.

Imaging the future of brain research

The first high definition imaging system, called Computed Axial Tomography (CAT scanning), was developed in the 1970s. It is an X-ray-based technology that was used, and still is, as a medical diagnostic tool to resolve the position of brain tumours in the brain for example. In the past 30 years more powerful imaging technologies have been developed that have the potential to associate different cognitive functions with different structures in the brain. These techniques include most notably Positron Emission Tomography and Magnetic Resonance Imaging.

When PET is used to link function to structure, increases in local blood flow and glucose consumption associated with increased neuronal activity are measured. A radioactive isotope, of glucose for instance, is injected into the blood stream and the high-energy photons that fly off in exactly opposite directions from the site of an emitting isotope are detected by an array of detectors that encircle the head. The detectors facing one another on opposite sides of the head will simultaneously detect the two photons generated from the same place within the brain. By the integration of simultaneous photon detection in the array, the source of the isotope can be calculated. In this way a computer builds an image of the structures that contain the isotope. In other applications of PET, the radioactive label is attached to molecules that bind to particular receptors, thus revealing the distribution of neurotransmitter systems receptors in the brain, for example.

A more sensitive technique, importantly that does not involve radioactive tracers, is Magnetic Resonance Imaging or MRI. Briefly the technique involves the pulsing of a strong external magnetic field, which evokes transient magnetic responses within the brain. The evoked magnetic signals are used to compute 2D and 3D images of the brain's structure. This technique can be used for purely structural studies, as it was in the experiments on London taxi drivers that showed they have a larger than expected hippocampus (see Chapter 6). But in its most interesting experimental application it provides images of the brain in action. When used to reveal active regions of the brain involved in particular functions, the technique is known as functional MRI, or fMRI for short.

To understand how fMRI works, and to appreciate its limitations, it is important to realize that it does not image the electrical activity of neurons directly. It monitors the indirect consequence of their activity. When a region of the brain is actively working, more neurons in that region will require more glucose and oxygen. This is a consequence of two interesting facts. First, it seems neurons only store enough energy for the briefest of bouts of activity. If neurons are active long enough, they need refuelling to enable them to produce the energy storage molecule ATP required to recharge their batteries (see Chapter 3). An active brain region therefore may have a significantly higher metabolic demand for oxygen and glucose than a quiescent region.

A simple solution to this problem would be to pump more blood into the active brain, much in the same way that a muscle is supplied with more blood when exercised vigorously. However unlike a muscle, which becomes engorged with blood and swells when exercised, the brain is confined by the skull and cannot be allowed to swell significantly. The solution to this tricky problem is to maintain a constant overall blood-volume in the brain and to arrange for blood to be diverted preferentially to active regions. Blood is diverted by the ability of blood vessels in the brain to dilate in response to signals coming from nearby active neurons. Dilation reduces resistance to blood flow, thereby increasing the supply of blood to the region of elevated neuronal activity.

We are not really sure how the blood vessels 'know' that nearby neurons are hyperactive. It is likely however that the signal for blood vessel dilation is the gas nitric oxide (NO), because NO causes the relaxation of muscle cells in the walls of blood vessels. It is thought that NO-producing neurons sense increased activity of nearby neurons and respond by producing NO in the same region – thus coupling increased neural activity to increased blood flow in that region.

In detecting regions of increased blood flow, fMRI recognizes the different magnetic signatures of oxygenated and deoxygenated haemoglobin. When neurons in a brain region are sufficiently active for long enough, blood in their vicinity becomes oxygen depleted. This is followed by an increased flow of oxygenated blood to that region; quite literally there is a local blushing of the brain. The fMRI technique is responsive to the blushing and indirectly assigns increased neural activity to that region at a spatial resolution of just a few cubic millimetres. It is in this way that we now have a far more fine-grained functional map of the brain than was previously possible. Bold claims are now being made about complex cognitive functions: where in the brain we recognize faces and words, where executive functions are carried out, where false memories are located, and so on.

Chapter 3
Signalling in the brain: getting connected

The problem of connection, the sending of information effectively around the nervous system, arises because signals must be communicated undistorted over the length of the body, which might be a very large distance indeed, in the case of the blue whale for example. Coupled to this is the fact that, in an unforgiving world, animals must react quickly to be an effective predator or so as to avoid being eaten. So the basic requirements of signalling coded information in the nervous system are that the signals have to be routed correctly and sent reliably over long distances *as rapidly as possible*.

In order to achieve this neurons convey and encode information electrically. Brief electrical pulses (lasting a few thousandths of a second), known as action potentials or nerve impulses, travel along biological cables (axons) that extend from the cell bodies of neurons to connect their input to their outputs with other neurons. Compared to the speed of electrical information traffic along the wires in a computer (close to the speed of light), conduction velocities of impulses in the brain are slow, about 120 metres per second in the fastest conducting axons. When they reach the terminals of axons, impulses trigger the release of chemical signals that are able to initiate or suppress electrical signals in other neurons. In this way neurons transmit information from one to another by an alternating chain of electrical and chemical signals.

The chemical signals are released at specialized sites called synapses, at which the chemical signals (neurotransmitters) pass across a very narrow gap separating two neurons. Released neurotransmitter molecules work by binding to and thereby activating specialized receptor molecules located on the surface of the receiving neuron on the other side of the synapse.

An activated receptor causes a brief electrical response, called a synaptic potential, in the receiving neuron. These potentials may be either inhibitory or excitatory depending on whether the voltage in the receiving neuron becomes more negative (inhibitory or hyperpolarizing) or less negative (excitatory or depolarizing). Inhibitory potentials make the receiving neuron less likely to fire a nerve impulse. Excitatory potentials increase that probability. A 'decision' to produce nerve impulses is therefore made through the summation of all of the inhibitory and excitatory potentials impinging on a neuron. Once a critical threshold voltage is reached by this summation, nerve impulses will be generated. The more the excitation, the higher will be the frequency of the impulse train. An important way that information is coded in the brain is by the impulse frequency (number of impulses or action potentials per second) and by the pattern of impulses. Nerve impulses travel rapidly along the axon, feeding information to many other neurons where the process of neurotransmitter release and chemical communication is repeated.

Neurons may receive chemical signals from hundreds of other neurons through a thousand or more synapses on their surfaces, each having some influence on the 'decision' to fire a nerve impulse and on the firing rate. The complexity of the resulting signalling network in the brain is almost unimaginable: one hundred billion neurons each with one thousand synapses, producing a machine with one hundred trillion interconnections! If you started to count them at one per second you would still be counting 30 million years from now!

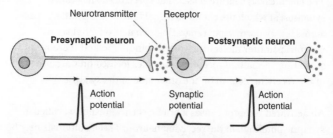

Neurotransmitter   Receptor

Presynaptic neuron   **Postsynaptic neuron**

Action   Synaptic   Action
potential   potential   potential

3. **Neuron-to-neuron communication. An electrical action potential or nerve impulse travels at speeds up to 120 metres per second along the axon of the presynaptic neuron. When it reaches the synapse the impulse causes neurotransmitter molecules to be released. Receptor molecules react to the neurotransmitter molecules causing the postsynaptic neuron to be either excited (illustrated) or inhibited. An inhibitory synaptic potential would dip below the resting potential, making the postsynaptic neuron less likely to fire an action potential**

Physics and the problem of electrical signalling

When a neuron is inactive or at rest there exists a stable negative voltage across the membrane of about −70mv, known as the resting potential. When excited by another neuron, or in the case of a sensory receptor cell by a sensory stimulus, the neuron may generate a train of action potentials. Nerve impulses attain a positive voltage of about +50mv before returning to the resting potential. So the total voltage excursion of a nerve impulse is about 120mv or 0.12 volts.

We need now to understand something about how these electrical impulses are generated and propagated along axons in the wet, salty, and gelatinous medium that is the brain: a very unsuitable environment for an electrical signalling system. The problem is made even more difficult by the dreadful electrical properties of axons. Axons are very poor conductors of electricity, so bad in fact that over relatively short distances, far less than a typical axon's length, most of the original signal will leak away into the salty surroundings. This inescapable problem is a consequence of the way the laws of physics apply to the flow of electricity in electrical cables immersed in salty water.

These laws were first formulated by the British scientist Lord Kelvin (1824–1907) who figured out how to send telegraphic information across the Atlantic Ocean through a submarine cable. Lord Kelvin defined a parameter called the 'length constant', which allows us to compare how good different types of cable are at transmitting electrical signals over a distance. A length constant is the distance over which about two-thirds of the electrical signal's amplitude will be lost and its value can vary enormously. For example, the length constant of a submarine cable is a few tens of miles. This means it is not possible simply to lay a cable across the Atlantic and expect an electrical signal injected at one end to appear at the other end undiminished, several thousands of kilometres away.

For a submarine cable, the length constant is a small fraction of the distance over which information must be sent and the same is true for biological cables, axons. So in a similarly salty environment both submarine cables and axons must detect a failing electrical signal and boost it back to its original strength before sending it on its way again. In submarine cables booster amplifiers placed at regular intervals achieve this, and axons solve the problem in a rather similar way. But how, using the unlikely ingredients of a few proteins, fats, some smaller organic molecules, and plenty of salty water, can nerve cells make a battery-powered amplifier?

The brain's batteries and impulses

The brain is a major consumer of bodily energy. While it is only 2 per cent of our body weight, it consumes 20 per cent of our energy and moreover 80 per cent of the brain's energy consumption is devoted to a single task: producing biological batteries, the power source of the amplifiers of electrical signals in axons.

Neurons in fact create two batteries. One has a value of about 50mv and faces inwards (positive pole inside) and the other has a value of about 70mv and faces outwards (positive pole outside). If the 70mv battery is turned ON and the 50mv battery OFF, the inside of the neuron will have a potential of –70mv. On the other hand if we now turn OFF the 70mv battery and turn ON the 50mv battery, then the inside will be positive by the value of the inward facing battery: i.e. +50mv. At the peak of an action potential the membrane voltage reaches about +50 mv before returning within a thousandth of a second to its resting value of about –70 mv. It is as if the action potential results from the rapid switching ON and OFF of the batteries in a well-defined sequence. This sequence of switching is initiated by a positive shift of the voltage across the membrane. If the positive change in voltage reaches a critical threshold value, the +50mv battery is turned on and a nerve impulse is initiated.

These batteries are 'charged up' by proteins that literally pump two positively charged ions in opposite directions across the membrane of the neuron. The process requires energy to be expended and this is achieved by the ability of molecular-scale pumps to couple the expenditure of metabolic energy to the movement of ions. Sodium ions are pumped out of the neuron whilst potassium ions are pumped in. These ions are derived from sodium chloride (table salt) and potassium chloride that are dissolved in the fluid surrounding all of our cells, providing a salt-water environment for them that is similar to the composition of the sea water in which cellular life had its origins. The pumping creates an imbalance between the inside and outside concentrations of the two ions. Sodium ions are maintained at about tenfold higher concentration outside than inside the neuron and approximately the reverse situation exists for potassium. These concentration gradients, in the absence of barriers, would result in sodium entering and potassium leaving the neuron.

Highly specialized protein molecules called ion channels restrict this passage of sodium and potassium into and out of the neuron by acting as molecular gatekeepers. Mobile parts of the molecule, 'gates', open and close in an orderly sequence. This molecular machinery enables the membrane to control the switching on and off of the sodium and potassium batteries. Each potassium channel has a single gate, known as the activation gate because when opened the flow of potassium is activated. The sodium channel is more complicated and has two gates, the activation gate and an inactivation gate. When the sodium activation gates are open sodium floods into the neuron due to the concentration gradient. This is equivalent to turning ON the 50mv sodium battery, making the inside of the neuron reach its maximum positive potential of +50mv at the peak of the nerve impulse. When the potassium gates open, equivalent to turning ON the −70mv battery, potassium flows out.

Now let's consider how nerve cells generate an electrical impulse from about −70mv to about +50mv and back in a few milliseconds. At the resting potential of about −70mv the sodium battery is switched off, so sodium flow is virtually entirely blocked because, although the inactivation gates are open, the activation gates are closed. The potassium battery is partly on because a small proportion of the potassium channel gates are open and some potassium is therefore free to flow out of the neuron, leaving the inside negative. To move the voltage to +50mv the activation gates for the inward flow of sodium must be opened. Then, to return to the resting potential the sodium gates must be closed and the potassium battery fully switched on, so that potassium flows out. The sequence of opening and closing during a nerve impulse is shown in Figure 4.

In order to understand these crucial parts of the signalling story we need know what causes the molecular-scale gates to open and close. The answer is that they are sensitive to the voltage across the membrane, allowing the detection of small changes in voltage and their amplification into discrete pulses of much greater amplitude. But how can these channel proteins sense and respond to the

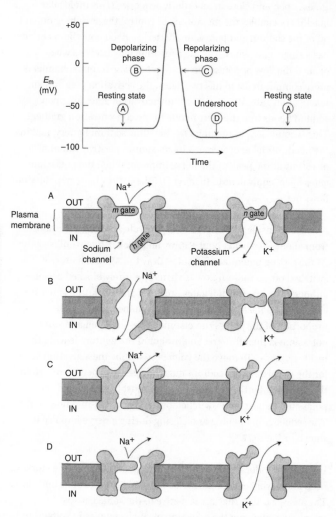

4. **Action potential and ion channels.** This illustrates how the molecular ion gates and channels in the nerve cell membrane (plasma membrane) behave at different stages (A to D) of the action potential

voltage across the membrane? It would seem that the proteins would have to be very sensitive indeed to changes in voltage – after all, a change of just a few thousandths of a volt across the membrane can be sufficient to trigger the opening of a channel gate.

Take a channel's eye view of the fluctuating membrane voltage however and we get a more realistic impression of the strength of the electrical forces acting on them. The membrane is exceedingly thin (about one millionth of a centimetre) and the total voltage change across this membrane during an action potential is 0.12 volts. If we take the thinness of the membrane into account, the fluctuation experienced by the protein is an enormous 120,000 volts per centimetre. As the gates of the ion channels are themselves electrically charged, they will be moved by the change in the electrical forces across the membrane. It is this movement of the ion gates that is the key to understanding how a small electrical excitation is amplified into a full-blown nerve impulse. The first gates to respond to an excitation are the ones preventing the entry of sodium. A very small excitation will open a few of these gates, allowing the inflow of sodium. This will cause the voltage to become even more positive, thus opening more sodium gates. If enough sodium gates are opened we quickly enter a positive feedback loop, leading inexorably to the turning on of the +50mv sodium battery at the peak of the nerve impulse. The voltage returns to its resting voltage by the delayed closure of the sodium inactivation gates and by the delayed opening of the potassium gates.

Speed is important

Biological cables are inherently slow conductors of signals because the nerve impulse depends on the movement of ions across a membrane rather than the displacement of electrons along a wire. Higher transmission speed can be achieved by improving the insulation of the axon membrane and by increasing the electrical conductivity of the axon's core. The latter can be achieved simply by increasing the axon's diameter. The fatter the axon the faster the transmission; for speed you need giant axons. Unfortunately this solution has significant practical drawbacks. The relationship between axon diameter and conduction speed is unfavourable – to double the speed you must quadruple the diameter (conduction velocity is proportional to the square root of the axon diameter). So to obtain significant gains in speed we would have to produce axons of gigantic girth. A related drawback is that a brain would contain fast components, but inevitably there would be fewer of them. Evolving high performance brains depended in part on the miniaturization of the brain's components and on getting as many fast neurons as possible packed into a small volume. For this, evolutionary selection pressure did not favour giant neurons.

Nonetheless, giant axons certainly do exist in brains. There are many examples in the nervous systems of invertebrate and lower vertebrates, where they tend to be involved in initiating very rapid responses such as escape reactions. An example of particular note is the giant axon of the squid, which can be up to 1 mm in diameter and transmits nerve impulses from the brain to the body musculature at several metres per second. This axon activates the animal's emergency escape behaviour, which requires the rapid contraction of the mantel cavity causing an explosive expulsion of water and a 'jet propelled' escape. In the 1940s the enormous dimensions of this particular axon attracted the attention of two British physiologists, Alan Lloyd Hodgkin and Andrew Fielding Huxley. They conducted a series of elegant experiments on the nerve impulse, using the size of the squid's giant axon to their advantage. Their experiments led to the discovery of voltage-sensitive sodium and potassium flow and to the ionic theory of the action potential described above. The Hodgkin and Huxley account of the action potential in the squid axon was to earn them a share of the Nobel Prize for Physiology and Medicine in 1963, not least because the principles and mechanisms uncovered in the squid were universal – explaining even how our axons transmit electrical signals. It seems a little unfair on the squid that there is no formal acknowledgement of its contribution to one of the most outstanding achievements of 20th-century science.

Transmission speeds in excess of 100 metres per second are possible by improving the axon's insulation with a multilayered Swiss-roll-like wrapping called myelin. At approximately 1 mm intervals the myelin wrapping is interrupted by gaps known as nodes of Ranvier where the axonal membrane is exposed. Voltage sensitive sodium channels are concentrated at the nodes and the nerve impulse seems to jump from node to node with negligible delay. The autoimmune disease known as multiple sclerosis (MS) cruelly highlights the importance of myelin in normal brain and bodily function. In MS the body's immune system damages the myelin and the ability of axons to conduct action potentials is disrupted. This produces various symptoms including unsteady movements of the limbs, blurred vision, abnormal eye movements, loss of coordination, slow word recall, and forgetfulness.

Myelin is produced by glia, cells in the nervous system that outnumber neurons at least tenfold. There are many other functions of glial cells; for example, the microglia are able to move around the brain, consuming dead cellular debris as they go. Other glial cells can alter the way neurons interact with one another, suggesting that the idea that glia merely provide supportive roles for neurons is wrong. Indeed recent experiments have shown that glial cells can detect changes in the voltage across their membranes and are responsive to chemical signals from neurons. Others are able physically to cover or uncover regions of communication between neurons, suggesting they can direct information traffic between different parts of the brain. If, as now seems probable, the neurons and glial cells are together essential for information processing, then by considering only the neurons we have vastly underestimated the complexity of the brain machine.

From neuron to neuron

Neuron to neuron communication occurs at specialized points of contact between nerve cells called synapses and there is perhaps in excess of 100 trillion of them in the human brain. Synaptic communications are essentially private, in the sense that a single synapse allows one neuron to speak to just one other. The cell bodies of communicating neurons need not be close to one another because neurons can reach out with long connecting processes. Synapses however are not the sole means of between-neuron communication and an important distinction can be drawn between point-to-point information transmission mediated by them (the brain's wiring diagram) and a more global form of non-synaptic information transmission (for which wireless broadcasting is a better analogy).

The point-to-point nature of synaptic communication between the wire-like fibrous extensions of neurons is reminiscent of an electronic circuit. Indeed the synaptic 'wiring diagram' of connections required for a particular brain function may be referred to as the neural 'circuit' for that function. Synapses require two neurons to cooperate in the formation of a small region of either direct contact (an electrical synapse) or very close apposition (a chemical synapse). Where there is direct contact, electrical signals pass with almost no delay from one neuron to another through protein pores that perforate the membranes of both neurons at the point of contact. Usually electrical synapses are bi-directional, electricity being able to pass equally well in both directions. Electrical synapses can be thought of as soldered joints in an electronic circuit; they are highly reliable connections and invariant in their operation, neither adding to nor subtracting from the signal passing between components. The speed and reliability of electrical synapses is exploited in neural circuits required for the activation of a flight response. In an escape behaviour there is no time for complicated information processing; escape must be executed as quickly and reliably as possible and this is a job ideally

38

suited to the simple, slavish, and fast properties of electrical synapses. The next time you unsuccessfully try to swat a fly your failure will be due to the speed of transmission of visual information (about you) passing through electrical synapses in the escaping fly's brain.

At a typical chemical synapse a narrow gap or cleft between two communicating neurons makes the direct exchange of electrical or chemical signals impossible. For information to be transmitted across the gap the electrical activity of a neuron must cause the release of a chemical message that diffuses across the synaptic cleft to the receiving neuron. The synaptic machinery allowing electrical activity in the signalling neuron to be coupled to the release of neurotransmitter is highly complex and specialized, as are the mechanisms that capture the chemical message and initiate responses in the receiving neuron. This means that the two sides of a chemical synapse are specialized for either sending or for receiving chemical messengers but not both. Signals therefore pass in one direction only, from the pre-synaptic to the post-synaptic neuron. The pre-synaptic side is specialized for the synthesis, storage, and release of a neurotransmitter. On the post-synaptic side the chemical message is recognized and converted into an electrical signal. Usually chemical synapses occur between the axon terminations of the transmitting neuron and the dendrites or cell body of the receiving neuron.

The simplest form of synaptic transmission involves an ion channel receptor (an ionotropic receptor) that is opened by the binding of a neurotransmitter. These mediate a direct and rapid coupling between neurotransmitter binding and the generation of a brief electrical signal in the post-synaptic neuron. There is another important category of 'indirect' neurotransmitter receptors (metabotropic receptors): the signal they generate is biochemical rather than electrical. When a neurotransmitter binds to an indirect receptor it activates a complex cascade of biochemical or metabolic events in the post-synaptic neuron, mediated by special enzymes that cause the synthesis of signalling molecules called second messengers.

Primary messengers are the neurotransmitters, which transmit information from neuron to neuron. Second messengers are the neuron's internal messenger molecules. It is through their action that the physiological properties of neurons and their synapses can be altered, either briefly or for extended periods of time. Second messengers are even involved in transmitting information from the synapse to the neuron's nucleus where they initiate long-term changes in the pattern of gene expression and protein synthesis that can in turn cause changes in the strength of synapses. It is in the action of second messengers therefore that we must seek a mechanism for the changes in the strength of synapses that accompany the process of memory formation in the brain (see Chapter 6).

The electrical circuit, 'wiring diagram', analogy is a compelling and useful one, but neurons can communicate without synapses. By the release of freely diffusing messenger molecules, such as the gas nitric oxide, some neurons broadcast information through volumes of the brain; communicating with many other neurons within the affected volume, without the need to be directly connected to all of them by synapses. Neurons may participate in both modes of transmission simultaneously. Indeed it may not be possible to understand how a function is performed without knowing both the synaptic wiring diagram of its neural circuit *and* how the circuit is influenced by signals being broadcast into it from elsewhere.

Putting this all together

In this chapter we have examined in some detail the cellular and molecular mechanisms of the most basic of brain functions – the ability of the brain's component cells to communicate with one another. What emerges is a picture of bewildering complexity in which it is not easy to see the wood for the trees. So let us stand back and imagine our brain with its hundreds of trillions of synaptic connections. Each synapse is potentially a unique computational unit with its own molecular tool kit, history, memory, and function. The neurons and their synapses are in a constant state of flux – the connections are dynamic, changing their strength, size, and location; being formed and unformed. Every second, millions of electrical impulses course along the fine fibrous extensions of the neurons, carrying electrical and chemical messages through a gelatinous interconnected circuitry that is more complex by far than that of any computer. If the interconnecting fibres in just one cubic millimetre of cortical grey matter were unravelled and laid end to end, they would form a strand 5 km (about 3 miles) long! If the connections in the whole brain were unravelled, the strand would be long enough to encircle the earth twice – such is the phenomenal interconnectivity of the brain. And this is only part of the story because the neurons and their connections make up a very small fraction of the brain's cellular machinery. There are as many as 100 glial cells for each nerve cell and we are only beginning to understand just how important they are, not simply carrying out housekeeping jobs but participating in the brain's computations, in among other ways, by regulating synaptic transmission.

This then – the neurons and their connections and their history, their companion glial cells, the multitude of chemical messengers and receptors – is basically all there is to the brain. We are far from understanding how it works as a whole but there is nothing more, no magic, no additional components to account for every thought, each perception and emotion, all of our memories, our personality, fears, loves, and curiosities.

Chapter 4
From the Big Bang to the big brain

Early evolution of the nervous system

Astronomers tell us that our universe began with a bang, in fact a Big Bang. Today in our small corner of this universe, some 14 billion years later, physical entities capable of reflecting on their place in this universe have somehow come to exist. It is safe to assume that brains did not simply spring into existence suddenly from nowhere, but how and by what route were brains created? The answer is that, in common with all other manifestations of life, the brain is the result of the haphazard and perilous process of evolution by natural selection. It did not happen overnight.

Our planet Earth came into existence about 4.5 billion years ago. In the beginning there was no life but within a billion years or so, the pre-biotic chemistry of life got started and the first primitive organisms appeared. Thus began the process of organic evolution leading to our present-day over-sized human brains. It was a process that would require three and a half thousand million years to complete.

As far as we know we are the first self-aware inhabitants of Earth, and almost certainly the first to question our origins and place in this strange universe. Today we are on the threshold of manned exploration and exploitation of other planets in our solar system and perhaps beyond. More than anything else it is our inquisitive and irrepressibly self-confident brains that have driven this quest for understanding and allowed all of this to happen.

Insight into the process by which our brains came to exist and to acquire their remarkable abilities can be gained by studying animals far simpler than us. Most animals have a nervous system and some form of brain, which is simply a concentration of nerve cells – usually sensibly placed at the front end. While we may be the only species endowed with a brain that bothers to think about itself, even this must have originated in the task of sensing and responding to the environment. These are the most basic functions of the nervous system – providing animals with the ability to detect salient features of their changing surroundings and to respond appropriately. While the brain has elaborated the art of sensing and responding, this ability is by no means exclusive to it. It is of almost unimaginable antiquity, predating the nervous system by a considerable margin, and can be traced to the earliest steps in the origin of life, crucially to the evolution of the very first biological cell.

Early cells had an aquatic existence and soon acquired the ability to move. Single cells swim using a variety of means including the lashing of whip-like flagella and the coordinated waving of many shorter 'hairs' called cilia. Other unicellular organisms can creep along by extending and retracting 'feet' or pseudopodia from the body of the cell. Importantly, movement enabled the early unicellular creatures to explore and exploit more of their world and its resources. When the ability to move was coupled with the ability to sense, movement could be directed to resource-enriched regions and individuals doing this most effectively reproduced more and prospered.

So even a single free-living cell can behave adaptively, can orient, and move 'intelligently' in response to environmental stimuli, combining all of the sensing and acting functions necessary for survival without a nervous system. This can be seen in modern-day unicellular organisms such as the ciliated protozoan *Paramecium*, which has a rich repertoire of orientation behaviours. They can sense and then swim towards their major food source – decaying organic matter. *Paramecium* also has a primitive touch sense enabling it to navigate around obstacles after colliding with them. This involves reversing the direction of swimming and turning away from the obstacle before proceeding in the forward direction. This behaviour is mediated by changes in the voltage across the cell membrane associated with the influx and efflux of calcium and potassium ions. Thus mechanical stimuli evoke electrical potentials much like nerve impulses in neurons.

As we have seen, the molecular machinery of sensing and acting existed in unicellular organisms, long before the arrival of multi-cellular animals. But the ability to act on sensations was transformed when multi-cellular organisms evolved. Now cells could cooperate with one another, dividing between them different and highly specialized roles. Individual cells no longer had to perform each and every essential role; they could 'differentiate' functionally one from another. Thus was the stage set for the evolution of the nervous system – a collection of highly differentiated cells designed for sensing, analysing, storing, and transmitting information and for directing adaptive behaviour in the interests of the survival and reproduction of the whole organism. The toolkit required for chemical and electrical signalling on which the functioning of the nervous system depends was already available. The brain did not have to invent everything from scratch – it evolved by modifying and incorporating mechanisms pre-existing in brainless animals.

It is likely that the first animals to have true neurons had a nervous system consisting of a diffuse *nerve net* with little or no concentration of nerve cells in any particular part of the body. This distributed feature of the nervous system works well for radially symmetrical animals in which no particular part of the body is more

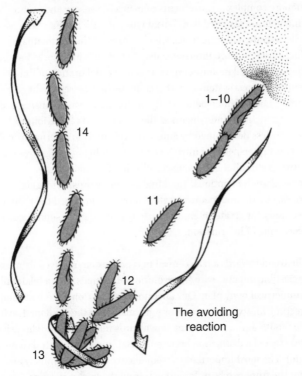

5. *Paramecium* avoidance behaviour. An animal consisting of just one cell can sense and respond to its world – without the need for a brain. However, the molecular mechanisms that underlie this simple avoidance behaviour are similar to those that underlie the electrical nerve impulse in the neurons of our own brains

or less likely than any other to encounter food or danger first. In its simplest state, the nerve net consists of sensory neurons, directly acting on contractile cells. Because these neurons must sense the outside environment they are derived from cells that make up the outer layer of the body, the ectoderm. Interestingly, our brains are derived in the embryo from ectodermal tissue that during the course of development becomes internalized.

45

In more complex arrangements of neurons, sensory and motor functions are assigned to different types of cells. Specialized sensory cells activate motor neurons, which innervate the contractile cells. There are few if any 'inter-neurons' – nerve cells interposed between the sensory and motor neurons. It is in the elaboration of the central nervous system in higher animals that we see the huge proliferation of inter-neurons. By mediating between sensing and motor functions, inter-neurons allow an animal's behaviour to become less determined by automatic reactions to external stimuli. In effect inter-neurons introduce the possibility of a cognitive gap between stimulus and response, allowing for intelligent consideration of options, 'thinking' in other words, before actions are executed. Inter-neuron proliferation also provided the numbers necessary for greater memory capacity and for more sophisticated processing of information.

The trend towards a true central nervous system received its most irresistible impetus with the evolution of animals with a bilaterally symmetrical body plan. Our ancestors had an elongated body and creeping lifestyle, feeding on organic matter on the sea floor. Having the mouth at the front facing downwards made this lifestyle easier and created a distinction between dorsal (top side), ventral (bottom side). The most important consequence of bilateral symmetry is that the front can be differentiated from the back – in effect inventing the head end. As most bilaterally symmetrical animals move in the forward direction, it made sense to concentrate the senses and the central nervous system at the head end, a phenomenon known as 'cephalization'. After all, the front end will encounter opportunity, food, and danger first, explaining why the brain of most animals is at the front.

With the exception of the most primitive of bilateral animals, the body is divided lengthwise into a series of segments. This is most evident in annelid worms such as earthworms and leeches where the body consists of virtually identical segments. The segmentation of the body is reflected in the segmentation of the central nervous system. In worms and insects each body segment contains a central 'ganglion', a collection of nerve cells concerned with the sensory and motor functions of that body segment. The ganglia are connected to one another by paired longitudinal 'connectives' containing the axons of nerve cells that communicate between ganglia. The ganglia thus form a 'nerve cord' running the length of the body. This ensures that the ganglia do not act independently and that the body segments cooperate with one another in the generation of coordinated behaviour.

In bilateral invertebrates the nerve cord is ventral to the alimentary canal or gut. This contrasts to the situation in the vertebrates, in which the spinal cord is dorsal, the gut lying ventral to it. You might imagine that the plans of the invertebrate and vertebrate nervous system are so fundamentally different that they must have very different evolutionary histories. But the vertebrates and invertebrates share more similarities than differences. Let's deal directly with the dorsal versus the ventral position of the central nervous system. During embryonic development, genes are expressed that determine the developmental programmes leading to specifically dorsal and ventral tissues. These genes are very similar in their DNA structure in invertebrate and vertebrate species, and they must therefore have derived from common ancestral genes. However, the genes in vertebrates that determine ventral tissues and organs are most closely related to the genes in invertebrates that specify dorsal. It seems that the only plausible evolutionary explanation for this apparent reversal of the functions of these genes is that something happened to one of our common ancestors that caused it to roll over, so that what was the ventral surface now faced upwards – thus becoming, by definition, dorsal.

What might have caused the hapless creature to turn over? One possibility is that a mutation occurred causing the mouth to move from its downward facing position to an upward facing position. Our bottom-grazing creature would be severely handicapped, unless of course it simply flipped over to bring its mutated mouth

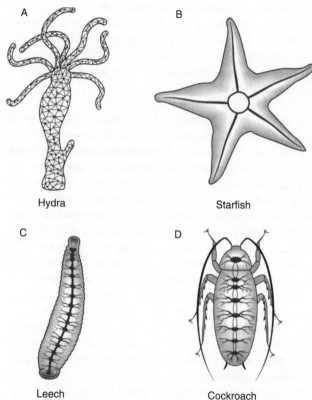

A

Hydra

B

Starfish

C

Leech

D

Cockroach

6. *Hydra,* Starfish, Worm and Insect: Simple nervous systems are diffuse networks of neurons (nerve nets) such as are found in modern day jellyfish and their relatives (*Hydra,* for example). The true central nervous system arises from the condensation of neurons into centres in which neurons are concentrated. In bilaterally symmetric animals such as worms and insects, the anterior end of the central nervous system becomes enlarged – a phenomenon known as cephalization. Cephalization resulted in the evolution of a true brain, located in the head. In animals with radial symmetry, such as the starfish, there is no head and thus no true brain

back to the preferred downward facing position. Now however the nervous system lies ventral to the gut just as it does in all of this creature's descendants – the vast majority of invertebrate animals. So what was ventral becomes dorsal and vice versa.

Overview of the human nervous system

The human brain has a confusing and complicated structural organization that certainly would not win awards for design. Unlike the eye, you cannot tell just by looking at it what the brain's true purpose is and prior to the scientific era scholars can be excused for suggesting that the brain functioned to cool the blood. After all, the folded surface of the cerebral cortex is at least suggestive of a heat exchanger or radiator.

Much of the brain's structural complexity arises because its evolution has been less of an 'out with the old, in with the new' process, and more a case of 'on with the old, in with the new'. This has resulted in new structures being layered upon more primitive ones, which may retain their original functions albeit in the context of the new opportunities provided by the newly acquired ones. Therefore a proper understanding of the brain can only really be achieved in the context of its evolution. It is also helpful to consider how the structure of the brain arises during the course of its embryonic development.

The human brain is basically an elaborated fluid-filled tube, which is first formed in the embryo. The two major subdivisions of the central nervous system, the brain and the spinal cord, are derived from a strip of embryonic skin on the dorsal midline called the neural plate. About three weeks after conception the neural plate rolls up to form a groove, which eventually pinches off at the midline to create the neural tube. The dorsal ectoderm then closes over the neural tube, which now resides inside the embryo extending from one end to the other. Flanking the neural plate is a region of ectoderm called the neural crest. Cells of the neural crest

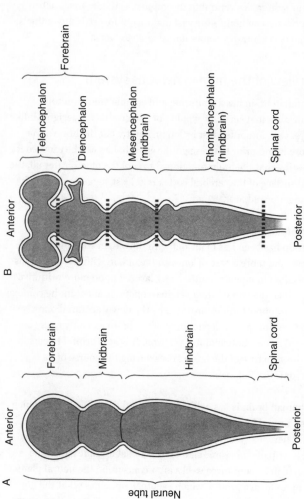

7. Three divisions of the brain early in development. At its anterior end the neural tube swells in three places, the forerunners of the fore- mid- and hindbrain (A). Later the swellings become further elaborated into the major subdivisions of the brain (B)

proliferate to form the peripheral nervous system, the autonomic system, and the sensory neurons of the dorsal roots of the spinal cord. The cells of the neural tube also proliferate, becoming the neurons and glial cells that form the brain and spinal cord. Initially the neural tube is uniform along its length, but as development proceeds, the rate of cell proliferation at the anterior end of the tube far exceeds the rate at the posterior end. Consequently the anterior end enlarges and later it will become the brain. The posterior end of the neural tube is destined to become the spinal cord.

At its anterior end the tube expands, forming three vesicles that will become the major divisions of the brain, the forebrain, midbrain, and hindbrain. These further subdivide to form the forerunners of the major component parts of the adult brain. For example, the anterior end of the forebrain balloons on each side, forming protrusions that will become the two cerebral hemispheres (the telencephalon). The protrusions on each side curl in a posterior direction before growing anteriorly, rather like a pair of ram's horns. Thus the most anterior part of the forebrain surrounds the midbrain. At the same time the embryonic mid- and hindbrain vesicles begin to differentiate and form all of the components of the brainstem.

From spinal cord to cerebral cortex

The spinal cord has a relatively simple structural organization: a central region of 'grey matter' containing synapses and the cell bodies of neurons and a surrounding 'white matter' consisting of the axons transmitting information up and down the cord. The spinal cord is segmental and at each segment there are two pairs of 'roots', one dorsal and one ventral, which connect the spinal cord to the body. The ventral roots contain the outgoing axons of motor neurons and the dorsal roots contain the incoming axons of sensory neurons. The cell bodies of the sensory neurons reside in swellings called dorsal root ganglia close to the spinal cord. Cell bodies of the motor neurons are found in the ventral grey matter, clustered

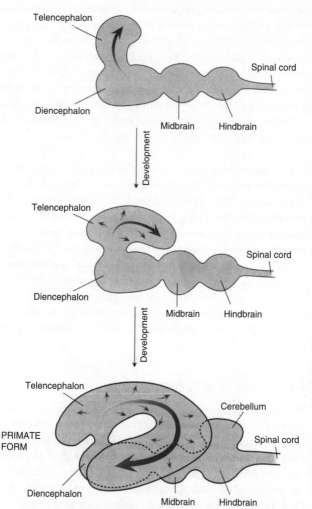

8. Development of the forebrain. During the embryonic development of the mammalian brain the most anterior part of the forebrain, the telencephalon, enlarges disproportionately. In primates, the telencephalon enlarges by curling round posteriorly and then anteriorly, eventually completely surrounding the rest of the forebrain and the midbrain

together in functionally related groups. Thus motor neurons that innervate a given muscle are grouped together and motor neurons of the extremities are found laterally in the cord, whereas those innervating trunk muscles are more centrally located. This grouping by function simplifies the task of activating groups of muscles sequentially to produce coordinated movements. Interneurons in the spinal cord connect the sensory input to the motor output and provide the neural circuits that underlie simple reflex behaviours such as the familiar knee jerk reflex.

The three divisions of the brain can be thought of as a hierarchy in which the forebrain controls the midbrain, which controls the hindbrain. The brainstem (mid- and hindbrain) is concerned with essential but non-cognitive bodily functions such as breathing, the regulation of blood flow, and the coordination of locomotion. Basic processing of sensory information is also performed by the midbrain structures, but more complex processing occurs when this partly processed information is distributed up the hierarchy to the forebrain. The forebrain can be regarded as the executive centre, which considers sensory information of all kinds and formulates commands, decisions, and judgements based on the sensory information and on experience. The increased complexity and flexibility of our behaviour can be attributed to increased cephalization – the acquisition of new neural functions associated with the most anterior parts of the brain. This is reflected in the increase in the relative size of the forebrain, which in fish, amphibians, and reptiles is a very minor part of the brain, but which in mammals is much larger. It becomes so large in humans that it will not fit into the skull without being folded into itself, forming the characteristic convolutions of the cerebral cortex.

The hindbrain consists of the medulla, pons, and cerebellum. The pons, medulla, and various divisions of the midbrain, described below, are referred to as the 'brain stem'. A substantial amount of space in the medulla is occupied by bundles of ascending and descending axons, carrying information traffic between the brain

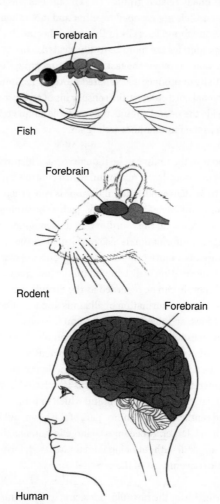

9. Cephalization. More and more resources are allocated to the most anterior part of the brain in vertebrate evolution. The relative size of the forebrain has increased most in evolutionary time. In hominid evolution the pre-frontal cortex (the most anterior part of the forebrain) tripled in size in just two million years

and the spinal cord. It is in the medulla that axon tracts descending from the cerebral cortex pass from the left to the right side, resulting in each hemisphere controlling movement on the opposite side of the body. Many visceral automatic functions, including breathing, heartbeat, and swallowing, are controlled by neural centres in the medulla. Just anterior to the medulla is the pons, a structure at the interface between the midbrain and hindbrain. It also has visceral functions and an important role in the control of facial expressions. It contains important sensory centres including the vestibular nuclei, which receive information about the orientation of the body with respect to gravity and acceleration.

The most complicated part of the hindbrain is the cerebellum, a structure specialized for the coordination of motor commands. In size the cerebellum is second only to the cerebral hemispheres. Placed over the gateway between the brain and spinal cord it is in a strategic position to oversee the performance of complex movements. The cerebellum has a very distinctive appearance, with a surface consisting of numerous ripples called folia separated by deep fissures. It is richly supplied with sensory information about the position and movements of the body and can encode and memorize information required for the execution of complex learnt skills. It is attached to the brain stem and connected to the rest of the brain by three pairs of axon tracts called peduncles that link it to the midbrain, the pons, and the medulla. The cerebellum has no direct connection to the cerebral cortex and while it also has a role in the control of movement, in contrast to the cortex each side of the cerebellum controls the same side of the body.

The midbrain consists of the substantia nigra, inferior colliculus, superior colliculus, and part of the reticular formation, which also extends into the medulla. The substantia nigra is intimately involved in the initiation and maintenance of voluntary movements. Damage to this part of the midbrain is linked with the symptoms of Parkinson's disease, a condition characterized by muscle tremor and a difficulty in initiating actions. The inferior colliculus is concerned with hearing and the superior colliculus is a centre for visual information processing and the generation of eye movements. The reticular formation has a primary role in the control and regulation of the arousal state of the brain.

The two major subdivisions of the forebrain are the telencephalon (cerebral cortex and the basal ganglia) and the evolutionarily older diencephalon (parts of the limbic system, the thalamus, and hypothalamus). In the diencephalon, deep in the brain, is a paired structure called the thalamus. This is a relay station for information on its way to the cerebral cortex coming from the visual, auditory, and body sensory systems. More ventrally, at the junction of the thalamus and the midbrain is the hypothalamus, a centre that in spite of its diminutive size is concerned with a wide range of important functions such as sex, emotion, the interpretation of smells, the regulation of body temperature, hunger, and thirst. It is the brain's link with the body's hormonal system and releases a number of hormones into its blood supply for distribution to the rest of the body.

The hypothalamus is usually included among a series of interrelated structures collectively called the limbic system. The term limbic refers to the parts of the forebrain that form a rim (*limbus* in Latin) around the bridge between the two cerebral hemispheres, the corpus callosum. This system includes the amygdala and the hippocampus that are, in an evolutionary sense, the oldest parts of the forebrain. The functions of these structures however changed in the course of evolution. In the lower vertebrates, reptiles for example, the amygdala is concerned with the sense of smell (olfaction), whereas in the human brain olfactory function is minimal and the area is thought to be mainly concerned with the emotions. Another example of evolutionary change of function is provided by the hippocampus. This structure in reptiles probably organizes behavioural responses to olfactory stimuli (such as either to flee or mate), but in mammals and man the hippocampus has a major role in the formation of memories. The cinglulate gyrus, another component of the limbic system, provides a connection between the limbic system and the cerebral cortex.

The anterior and most recently evolved part of the forebrain consists of the basal ganglia and the enveloping cerebral hemispheres. The basal ganglia lie hidden under the two hemispheres and consist of a cluster of three paired groups of neurons. Their role is to control and regulate voluntary movements initiated in the cerebral cortex. More than any other brain structure, it is the cerebral cortex that makes us human. Within the cortex plans are made, volitional behaviour is initiated, the neural machinery of language is located, and conscious perceptions are assembled from sensory information. It is the locus of all of our creative intelligence and imagination. If indeed we have free will, then it is in the cortex that its secret will be found.

The cerebral cortex is the convoluted surface of the two cerebral hemispheres and comprises a single folded sheet, about 2–4 mm thick. Information enters and leaves the cortex carried by about one million input–output neurons, but there are more than ten billion internal connections. The cortex therefore spends most of its time talking to other bits of itself. Extensive and pronounced infolding of the cerebral cortex allows a large surface to be accommodated by the skull. If the left and right cerebral cortices were ironed flat they would cover a surface of about 1.6 square metres, approximately four times the area covered by a chimpanzee's. A deep midline valley, the longitudinal fissure, divides the cortex into its left and right hemispheres. Both sides are subdivided into four principal lobes, which derive their names from the bones of the skull that lie over them. The frontal lobes are the largest, accounting for about 40 per cent of the cortex; the temporal, parietal, and occipital lobes account for about 20 per cent each. The ridges of the surface convolutions are called gyri and the valleys that separate them are called sulci, the deeper of which are called fissures. Superficially the left and right sides of the cerebral hemispheres are symmetrical in appearance and largely mirror one another functionally too. There are however important left–right differences concerning some cognitive tasks such as those required for language.

The deep longitudinal fissure that apparently separates the left from the right cortex along the midline conceals a major structure called the corpus callosum, which is of vital importance in bilaterally coordinated cortical function. It is the communications bridge between the cerebral hemispheres and consists of a tract of about one million axons, half of them originating from neurons in the right and half from neurons in the left cerebral cortex. The axons of the corpus callosum allow the left cortex to know what the right cortex is doing, has done, and might do next, and vice versa. If the corpus callosum is cut through, as it is infrequently in the treatment of intractable epilepsy, the two hemispheres can function independently. Following such operations, individuals referred to as 'split-brain' patients provided the definitive evidence that the two hemispheres differed in their roles in language. Split-brain patients have been able to name unseen objects held in the right hand. For this naming task the left hemisphere is used because sensory information from the right side of the body is processed by the left cerebral cortex. However, using the right cerebral cortex patients could not provide a verbal account of what was held in the left hand. These observations confirmed what had been assumed, namely that while both hemispheres have a conscious awareness of things, it is the left that expresses its awareness in words.

The convoluted surface of the human cortex can be divided into a number of functional regions, but the most basic and simple division is between areas serving sensory and motor functions. Sensory cortical areas are defined by the type of information that they receive, different areas being specialized to receive and process information coming from particular sensory organs and structures. For instance information from the eyes projects to the most posterior part of the occipital lobe known as the primary visual cortex. Information coming from the body and skin, called somatosensory information, projects to a strip of the parietal lobe known as the somatosensory cortex.

An important design principle of these sensory cortical areas is 'mapping'. The cortex constructs maps, spatial representations of the sensory world that is conveyed to it by sensory organs. The easiest one to understand is the map of the visual world, which is two-dimensional and formed initially in the eye, which projects an image of the outside world onto the retina. A neural representation of this map is preserved as it passes from the retina to the thalamus and then on to the primary visual cortex. The map is repeated several times in subdivisions of the cortex specialized for different aspects of visual perception. Left and right surfaces of the body are also mapped on the right and left cortical hemispheres respectively. They are called somatosensory maps and are found in the broad strips of cortex located just behind the central sulcus.

Movements of the body are controlled by the primary motor cortex, which is a mirror image of the sensory representation of the body surface described above. The left motor area controls the right side of the body and the right the left. The motor areas occupy the strips of cortical surface just in front of the central sulcus and there is a motor map, a map of muscles, which corresponds to the distorted representation of the body in the somatosensory maps.

None of these cortical maps are drawn to scale; instead they are variously distorted to reflect the amount of neural processing power devoted to different regions. This accounts for the grotesque appearance of the human form (Penfield's famous *homunculus*) that can be drawn from a translation of the body's sensory map into the human form.

Much of the cortex, often referred to as the 'association cortex', is not directly connected either with the motor control systems or with the initial stages of sensory information processing. Generally

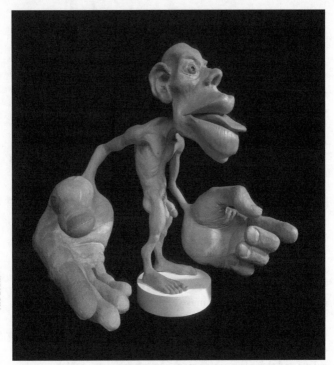

10. *Homunculus*: a distorted image of the human form reflects the differential allocation of cortical surface to sensory and motor functions of different parts of the body

the further removed from direct motor or sensory functions the cortex becomes, the less well can its function be defined.

How the human cortex became so big

If we trace the evolution of the human brain, the greatest and most rapid growth has occurred in the frontal lobes of the cortex, which accounts for some 40 per cent of the structure. In our nearest living relatives, the chimpanzees, the frontal cortex accounts for about 17 per cent. The evolutionary lines leading to modern humans and other living primates, including chimpanzees, diverged about 14 million years ago. The oldest bipedal hominids (3.9–2.5 million years ago) had a brain size ranging from 400 to 500 cc, only 100 cc or so larger than that of a chimpanzee. *Homo habilis* (2.5–2 million years ago), probably the first fabricator of stone tools, was slightly more cerebrally endowed with a brain size up to about 600 cc. So brain size had been increasing gradually, but relatively slowly, in primate evolution from 14 million to about 4 million years ago and in the early phase of hominid evolution up to about 2 million years ago. But over the course of the next 2 million years, brain size was almost to triple, with by far the greatest relative change occurring in the size of the frontal cortical lobes.

Neanderthal man, appearing first in Europe and western Asia, and modern man *Homo sapiens*, of African origin, are the most recent species in the hominid lineage. They appeared at approximately the same time: around 300,000 years ago for Neanderthal and 250,000 years ago for *Homo sapiens* and had roughly equivalent brain size, though in fact the Neanderthal average (1,500cc) is slightly greater than the human average (1,400 cc). Of course brains do not fossilize and we do not know what the relative size of the frontal cortex was in Neanderthal man. We do however know that in the course of human evolution much of the growth in brain size has been due to the explosion in the relative size of the frontal cortex. How did it get so big in such a brief period of evolutionary time; *why* has it become so conspicuously large? What is so special about the frontal cortex?

The frontal cortex is responsible for the processing of information from diverse and very widely separated regions of the rest of the cortex. It is in effect a complex integration centre that defines an individual's personality more than any other region of the brain. It creates an awareness of 'the self' in relation to the world and enables us to plan and execute actions into the future. Deficiencies and damage in the frontal cortex compromise the ability of an individual to make sensible predictions about the future consequences of events and actions in the present. Although intellectual power may be left unaltered, normal restraints on interpersonal discourse are seriously affected by frontal damage and one cannot help but conclude that much of what makes us human, civilized, and creative resides in the part of the brain that has grown so disproportionately in the course of our evolution.

Nobody really knows why the part of the brain that makes us unique should have evolved so rapidly; tripling in size in less than two million years. It certainly looks as though evolution entered a positive feedback loop in which natural selection favouring creative intelligence became linked to an ever more extravagant expression of that intelligence.

Although there is no watertight explanation for the runaway pace of evolutionary change that human brain development would seem to require, one of the more imaginative ideas is that our frontal brain is an ornament required for courtship display. According to this idea, the human brain is the product of the mutual preference of men and women for mating with partners who display unusually creative intelligence in the rituals of courtship. This can result in a form of natural selection called sexual selection. It depends on creativity in courtship and the large brain that it requires being heritable traits. If the larger brained individuals were genetically fitter specimens, which they may well have had to be to carry the burden of an enlarged brain, sexual selection can provide an explanation for the exaggerated size of the human cortex and runaway pace of human brain evolution.

A question that does not seem to be answered by the sexual selection hypothesis, and requiring further examination, is the reason for the late emergence of physical evidence of creative intelligence. Human beings, with brains equal in cubic and intellectual capacity to ours, first appeared in the fossil record more than 250,000 years ago. If their brains attained cleverness and creativity in the interests of seduction, why does significant proof of creative intelligence, such as cave paintings, not appear until just 35,000 years ago? This apparent discrepancy does not disprove the role of sexual selection in the brain's evolution, but suggests that it must be part of a more comprehensive explanation for our extraordinary brains. The truth is that we cannot yet explain why we enjoy exercising them in the creation and public display of music, art, poetry, and humour.

Chapter 5
Sensing, perceiving, and acting

Sensory perception's imperfections

Sensory information flowing into the brain fuels our perceptions, memories, intentions, and actions. Although we generally refer only to the five traditional senses – sight, touch, audition, taste, and smell – there are in fact many more. Other sensations include those of heat and cold, gravitation, acceleration, pain, etc. Moreover each of the traditional sensory modalities is a complex mix of distinctly different sub-senses. In the visual modality for example there is the ability to sense the motion, colour, form, brightness, texture, and contrast of objects.

The brain analyses primary sensations, transforming them into perceptions upon which informed decisions are made about future actions. Sensations however are just one contributory component to perception. It is possible to perceive what is not sensed, not to perceive what is sensed, and to construct more than one perception from the same sensations. Perceptions are not therefore strictly determined by sensations, nor are sensory perceptions linked to single modalities. Perceptions are the brain's educated guesses about what the combined senses are telling it, and as such they will almost always depend on interactions between different modalities. So while making a distinction between sensation and perception may seem academic, actually it is an important one.

This distinction can easily be appreciated by looking at the famous visual illusion based on a painting titled *My Wife and Mother-in-Law* by W. E. Hill. You will either see a young woman looking away or the profile of an old woman: two perceptions contained in the same picture. Once both have been perceived, it is possible to swap between the two at will. The sensory information falling on the retina is exactly the same for both, so there must be a top–down process determining how the perceptual system interprets the sensory input. In effect our brains impose different conscious perceptions on the same information registered by our sensory systems.

The importance for perception of the interaction between different senses is illustrated by the auditory-visual illusion known as the McGurk effect described by Harry McGurk and John MacDonald in an article called 'Hearing Lips and Seeing Voices'. Watching a video of a person repeating the syllable 'dah' three times followed by three repetitions of the syllable 'bah' can produce the illusion. If the soundtrack repeats the sound 'dah', irrespective of the syllable actually being mouthed, you hear both 'dah' and 'bah'. When you

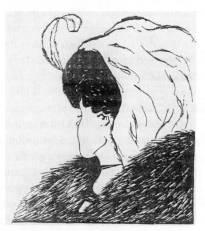

11. Two perceptions from one sensation

see the lips mouth 'bah' you hear 'bah' even though the sound entering your ear is in fact 'dah'. Your brain is trying to provide your consciousness with its best guess about what the senses are telling it. In this case there is a contradiction between what the eyes and ears are telling it to perceive. In this instance, the eyes have it.

Perceptual blindness is a striking example of the way the brain is highly selective in deciding which elements of the sensory information available to it are consciously perceived. A remarkable illustration of this is provided by a short video made by Daniel Simons and Christopher Chabris. The video shows a group of young people passing a basketball to each other. A person dressed in a gorilla suit walks into their midst, waves conspicuously into the camera, and then walks out of the scene. In advance of viewing the video, the audience is instructed to count the passes and then report their findings after the clip. Astonishingly, when I saw this demonstrated recently, about half the audience completely failed to notice the gorilla! But the invisible gorilla was there, its image entered the eyes of each viewer, impressed itself on their retinas, was sent to the thalamus from where it was relayed to the primary visual cortex. Where then did the proverbial 900lb gorilla go? It seems that the brain was so engaged in the counting task that it decided not to bother itself with generating a conscious perception of a gorilla, even though a substantial part of the brain's visual system was fully informed about its presence. So the gorilla was in effect airbrushed out of the visual perception.

How the brain might achieve such a feat of image manipulation is beyond our current understanding. The task must involve more than removing the visual information associated with the gorilla because the gorilla image is not replaced by a gorilla-shaped hole in vision. The space occupied by the gorilla is filled in appropriately with what would have been seen behind it had the gorilla not actually been there. Equally remarkable, those who witnessed the invisibility of the gorilla could not recall anything odd about their perception of the original video. Apparently there was no accessible memory trace left of the strange case of the disappearing gorilla. This example should make us sceptical about the veracity of eyewitness accounts where accuracy matters, in the reporting of crimes, for example.

Our human senses are impoverished when compared to those of other animals. A male moth when searching for a mate can for example respond to the 'smell' of individual molecules of the sexual attractant 'pheromone' which the female exudes into the air to lure a distant mate. Our eyes are sensitive to wavelengths in the electromagnetic spectrum between about 400 and 700 nanometres only. Many insects respond to shorter wavelengths, enabling them to use information contained in ultraviolet light. Other animals, such as some snakes, can 'see' the body heat of their prey using the long wavelengths of infrared radiation. Our hearing is similarly restricted to a narrow band of frequencies. At best we can hear sounds up to about 20 kHz, far short of the ultrasonic frequencies that bats use in echo locating obstacles and prey.

Perceiving the outer world

Open your eyes and you see the world around you apparently instantaneously, in colour and extraordinary temporal and spatial detail. Just a glance allows you to identify objects – their colour, shape, texture, size, location, and spatial relationship to one another are immediately apparent. If an object is moving with respect to you, you can instantly tell its direction of motion and estimate its speed, information that allows you to avoid colliding with it or to catch it. If you are in motion, you can see the flow of the visual world around you and extract information from it, enabling you to know your direction, estimate your speed, and simultaneously adjust both.

Seeing depends on the retina providing highly processed information on the quality and quantity of light captured by the rods and cones, the two systems of photoreceptors. The cones are highly concentrated at the fovea, an area of just one square millimetre at the back of the retina. This region is responsible for our high-acuity colour vision and could be rightly regarded as the most important square millimetre in your body. There are red, green, and blue sensitive cones and they provide information about the relative amounts of red, blue, and green light that the brain uses to 'colour in' an object. So the brain creates all the colours we can perceive by blending just three, much in the same way that an artist can mix any colour from just three pigments. As the cones are rather insensitive to light, colour vision is only possible in relatively bright light. In the majority of the retina surface, surrounding the fovea, the highly light-sensitive rod photoreceptors predominate, outnumbering the cones by some 10 to 1.

Light regulates the amount of neurotransmitter released by the rods and cones, which in turn regulates the electrical activity of neurons in the retina. These include the bipolar neurons that transmit information along the light-path and the horizontal and amacrine neurons that transmit information sideways in the retina – perpendicular to the light-path. The last neurons to be affected are retinal ganglion cells, the retina's output neurons whose axons form the optic nerves connecting the eye to the brain.

Your eyes operate over an enormous range of light intensities, from a starlit night to the brightest sunny day – perhaps a millionfold difference in luminance. This is achieved by a property of the photoreceptors called adaptation, which adjusts their sensitivity to match the average background light intensity. In very dim lighting the rod sensitivity is increased and in bright light their sensitivity is reduced. At any given level of sensitivity, the rods reliably report differences in light intensity within a narrow range above and below the average background level. The photoreceptors are therefore very sensitive to small changes in light intensity relative to the background but not to absolute intensity. If the overall background level of illumination were to change drastically, as it does when we enter a cinema on a bright sunny day, we are effectively blind until

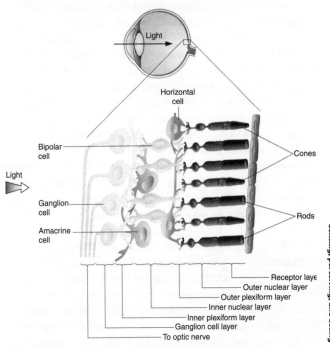

Light

Horizontal
cell

Bipolar
cell

Cones

Light

Ganglion
cell

Rods

Amacrine
cell

Receptor layer
Outer nuclear layer
Outer plexiform layer
Inner nuclear layer
Inner plexiform layer
Ganglion cell layer
To optic nerve

12. **Eye and retina. Light entering the eye passes through two layers of neurons in the retina before reaching the light-sensitive photoreceptors – the rods and cones. Information about the quality of the light is then passed back to the neurons, which integrate and transform it into a pattern of impulses for transmission to the brain by a million retinal ganglion cells**

our rod photoreceptors have adapted to the reduced intensity by increasing their sensitivity. Resetting sensitivity depends on the mobilization of biochemical mechanisms in the photoreceptors and can take a few minutes to complete for a very large change in light intensity. As a consequence of light adaptation, the brain is not informed about the absolute levels of brightness but about rather more useful information about local differences in brightness and contrast, regardless of the overall brightness.

Information travels to the brain from the eyes as trains of nerve impulses carried by the axons of the retinal ganglion cells. Each ganglion cell has a unique view on the visual world, called its receptive field. This is the small roughly circular region of the world, light from which can affect the electrical activity of a particular ganglion cell. There are roughly equal numbers of two different types of receptive fields of retinal ganglion cells, those that are excited by an increase in light intensity at the centre of their receptive field (ON centre ganglion cells) and those that are excited by a decrease in central intensity (OFF centre). By reporting an increased rate of firing for both ON centre and OFF centre receptive fields, a more reliable signal is generated than by reporting an ON response with an increased rate and an OFF response with a decreased rate from an already low firing frequency.

Vision is an active information acquisition process – the eyes dart about frenetically under the direction of the brain. As we have already discovered, clear vision is possible only when the fovea inspects a scene. This provides a very restricted window of clarity and so to generate the perception of a 'movie in the head' the eyes must be moved around. The eyes move speedily from one place to another where they dwell for a while, enabling your brain to take a high definition snapshot. From a number of these sequential snaps the brain builds the mind's eye picture of the outside world. The whole process is an active feedback loop in which the retina supplies information to the brain, which then makes an educated guess about what is out there and on this basis instructs the eyes to move, thereby changing the visual information being supplied. Multiple brain regions are required to perform all of the computational tasks that are necessary to convert information supplied by the eyes into the richness of perception that constitutes cinematic awareness of the visual world.

The pathway from the eye to the brain starts where the axons of the retinal ganglion cells exit the retina forming the optic nerve. At this point, called the optic disc, there are no photoreceptor cells to allow the ganglion cell axons to exit. Each optic disc is therefore insensitive to light and this produces the so-called 'blind spot' in the visual field of each eye. The optic nerves approach the brain along intercepting paths and meet at the base of the diencephalon at a crossing point called the optic chiasm, which directs the nerve fibres to their targets either on the same or opposite side of the brain. In humans, about 60 per cent of the ganglion cell axons in each optic nerve cross over in the chiasm, heading for targets on the opposite side of the brain, and the remaining 40 per cent are directed to brain targets on the same side. So, on the brain side of the chiasm the left and right bundles of ganglion cell axons, now called the optic tracts, include nerve fibres from both eyes.

Axons in the optic tracts have a number of targets in the brain, by far the most important for conscious visual perception being a region of the thalamus known as the lateral geniculate nucleus. Axons of retinal ganglion cells terminating in the lateral geniculate form synapses with other neurons and do not progress further into the brain. Neurons that have received visual information from the ganglion cells radiate out of the thalamus and go directly to the primary visual cortex (also referred to as the striate cortex or region V1).

It is important to realize that, in the lateral geniculate and in the cortex, the spatial relationships between neurons in the retina are maintained. These brain targets of eye-derived information thus contain map-like representations of visual space. Just as the eyes are paired, so too are the lateral geniculate nuclei and primary visual cortical areas. Visual information about the left side is mapped in the right lateral geniculate and the right visual cortex and the map of the right visual world is found in the left target regions. As the visual fields of both eyes overlap extensively, in the so-called binocular field, extensive regions of the left visual field are 'seen' by both left and right eyes and vice versa. The visual map in the right-hand side of the brain representing the left side of the

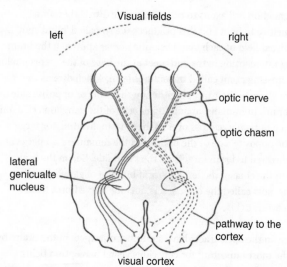

The Brain

13. **Optic pathway – eye to cortex.** Information about the left visual world is transmitted to the right side of the brain and *vice versa*. As the visual fields of the eyes overlap in the front, this division is achieved by sorting retinal ganglion cell axons according to whether they look at the left or the right visual fields. So some axons from the right eye go to the right side of the brain and others to the left. The sorting occurs in the optic chiasm. The retinal axons proceed to the lateral geniculate nuclei where the first synapses are formed with visual neurons in the brain

visual world therefore contains binocular regions that are constructed from information derived from both eyes.

In the lateral geniculate, visual inputs from the left and right eyes terminate in different layers so that neurons projecting to the cortex are excited by input from either the left or the right eye, but not by both. Geniculate neurons and the cortical neurons that they excite in cortical region V1 are therefore monocular. In subsequent stages of visual information processing in the cortex, inputs from the binocular fields of left and right eyes converge to produce neurons that have two receptive fields, one seen by the right eye and one by the left. Many such neurons are maximally excited when the neuronal pathway representing the same part of the visual world in both left and right eyes is activated. Other binocular neurons are excited when non-corresponding parts of the left and right visual fields are visually stimulated. As these binocular neurons report information about the same or nearby regions of the left and right visual field, they are likely to be important in generating the perception of depth when the same object is viewed using both eyes.

In the primary visual cortex simple details of the features of the visual field are analysed. The response properties and receptive fields of lateral geniculate neurons are similar to those of the retinal ganglion cells. But primary cortical neurons are relatively unresponsive to a small spot of increasing or decreasing brightness at the centre of their receptive field – very effective excitatory stimuli for geniculate and retinal neurons. The responses of lateral geniculate neurons are integrated in the cortex to produce high responsiveness to edges or bars with high light–dark contrast. Importantly, the primary cortical neurons respond best to bars or edges presented in a particular orientation angle within the receptive field. Not only do adjacent regions of the visual world project to adjacent neurons in the cortex, but the response properties of neurons that share the same position on the surface of the visual cortex also share qualitatively similar responses to visual stimuli. There is a systematic functional organization within and across the cortex. For example, neurons that are excited by the same optimal orientation are organized in vertical columns. Between adjacent orientation columns there is a gradual systematic shift of orientation preference such that all orientations around 360 degrees are represented every millimetre or so within the map of the visual world in the primary visual cortex. This ensures that every part of the cortical visual map contains neurons that are excited by all orientations.

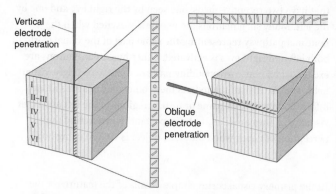

14. **Columnar organization in primary visual cortex. An electrode passing through the primary visual cortex vertically (left image) will encounter neurons with the same preferred orientation. An electrode moving horizontally or obliquely (right) will encounter a series of neurons whose preferred orientations change systematically. In layer IV of the cortex there are no orientation-selective neurons (denoted by circles)**

Partly processed visual information is now directed to a number of other regions of the cortex concerned with vision. In these extra-striatal visual areas, the visual maps of the external visual world are repeated several times. It seems the brain prefers to have individual neurons receiving information about adjacent objects in the outside world to be close to one another in the inner world of the cortex also. Here more complex aspects and features are assigned to the visual information.

As the integration and processing of visual information proceeds in the cortex, the response properties tend to become more complex. For example, a cortical neuron in the early stages of processing may respond only to an edge of a particular orientation presented in a particular part of the visual field. Many similar neurons therefore are required to represent in a distributed fashion the many orientations that make up the complexity of the visual world. At later stages in processing, neurons may respond to an edge of a

74

given orientation presented *anywhere* in the visual field. This is suggestive of a hierarchical organization of neuronal image processing and object recognition in the cortex, an idea which when taken to its logical conclusion led to the whimsical proposition that there is a neuron in your brain that only responds to your grandmother (the infamous grandmother cell hypothesis). But it is unlikely that visual perceptions are built by the serial processing of information from oriented bars, to depth, motion, adding colour, identifying object shape, object location, direction and rate of motion, texture, and so on. Each of these components of vision are processed separately and in different parts of the primary visual and extra-striatal visual cortex. It takes only a fraction of a second to recognize a familiar face or object, far less time than would be required if recognition depended on the processing of information serially, one feature at time. The problem with the notion of parallel processing, however, is that our most sophisticated understanding of vision derives from electrical recordings from single or just a few neurons. Important though these experiments are, they do not explain how all the disparate bits of information, each handled separately and in different parts of the brain, are bound together in visual recognition – of a flying banana for instance.

How neurons represent different visual perceptions, allowing for seemingly immediate recognition of familiar objects, remains one of the most important unanswered questions in neuroscience. Fascinating recent research on the recognition of famous people and buildings has however shed fresh perspective on the question. Currently on this question there exist two opposing hypotheses; divided by whether the encoding system is thought to be dispersed/ distributed or sparse. Most neuroscientists today believe that perceptions are dispersed over populations of neurons that require near simultaneous activation for the generation of visual percepts. According to this idea individual neurons in the population would respond to similar features contained in many recognizably different pictures. In other words, the activity of any individual neuron is not explicitly representative of a particular object. A minority of neuroscientists however claim that at the level of individual neurons the encoding system is explicit and highly selective. According to this idea the activity of visual recognition neurons is not distributed but 'sparse' – becoming increasingly so as the deciphering of an object proceeds. Thus for the sparseness camp, encoding involves the activation of fewer and fewer neurons as neuronal activity represents more and more selective combinations of object features. Those that argue for sparseness coding, however, are perhaps unfairly accused of believing in the simplistic notion that the brain has a separate neuron for every recognizable object, including one's grandmother.

Research shedding new light on this issue, and challenging the dismissive attitude to the sparseness camp, involved recording from individual neurons in the medial temporal lobe (MTL) of the cortex in human patients undergoing treatment for intractable epilepsy. Subjects were shown pictures of movie stars and famous buildings while the activity of single neurons in the MTL was recorded. One of the neurons responded when seven quite different pictures of the same actress, Jennifer Aniston, were shown. In an extraordinary display of selectivity and discrimination, however, the same neuron did not respond to pictures of Jennifer with her then husband Brad Pitt. These findings show that individual neurons can show a remarkable consistency of responsiveness across diverse images of the same object. In some instances a neuron would respond to the object and to the word representing the object. For example, one neuron responded selectively to different pictures of the Sydney Opera House and to the letter string 'Sydney Opera' but not to the letter string 'Eiffel Tower'. This study reported by Quiroga and colleagues supports the idea that, at late stages in the transformation of visual information into the recognition of the familiar, encoding is remarkably sparse. Also, 'invariance', the ability of our perceptual system to recognize the same object from any perspective, in light or shadow, can be detected in the activity of individual neurons. All of this however does not mean that the brain's visual recognition pathway does not depend on patterns of activity distributed across populations of neurons. It will nonetheless invigorate those who are not so dismissive of the 'grandmother cell' sparse coding idea – after all Jennifer Aniston may in time become a grandmother.

Although for conscious seeing the most important first pre-cortical destination for information from the eye is the lateral geniculate, there are other targets receiving information directly from the retina. Some retinal ganglion cell axons leave the optic tract before they reach the lateral geniculate nuclei and form a separate pathway that targets a region in the brain called the pretectum. Here they activate a reflex response to bright light that causes the constrictor muscles of the iris to contract, reducing the diameter of the pupil. The reflex is bilateral so both pupils are constricted at the same time, even if the bright light enters one eye only. Another important target for retinal ganglion cell axons is a region of the hypothalamus that is important in bodily functions that show a day/night or circadian rhythm.

The hypothalamic and pretectal targets do not require much spatial detail of the visual world, simply a representation of the overall light levels. For this reason these targets, in contrast to the lateral geniculate, do not receive retinal input organized as a spatial map. In fact some retinal ganglion cells that target them are capable of responding to light directly. They therefore do not need to be connected to either rod or cone photoreceptors.

Perceptions that drive actions

One group of retinal axons travel from the eye to a structure in the brain called the superior colliculus, with an important role in changing the direction of gaze from one object the brain finds interesting to another. For this task the superior colliculus needs to relate visual and motor maps to one another and its layered structure suggests how this is achieved. The superficial layer has a two-dimensional map of the visual world projected on to it, such that each point on the surface is excited by a visual stimulus in a particular part of the world. Deeper layers constitute motor maps corresponding to the visual sensory map residing directly above them. The deeper layers are effectively motor maps in the sense that activity in a particular site in the visual map lies immediately above the site on the motor layers that can generate a rapid saccadic eye movement precisely to the point in visual space that activated the visual map. The motor layers are responsible for initiating the bursts of nerve impulses in the motor neurons causing the direction of gaze to move very rapidly from one fixed point to another.

This organization ensures that when a potentially interesting object appears in the peripheral visual field, it will activate neurons in the corresponding part of the visual map. These neurons will be adjacent to (just above) the part of the motor map that can move the eyes, bringing the new object on to the fovea, allowing the brain to inspect it in greater detail. The fact that the layers are in register ensures that the shortest between-layer connections will produce the appropriate rotation of the eyes to fixate visually the new object.

This is a simple and elegant neural mechanism but it is not 'hard-wired'. If it were, every new object in our visual world would trigger an automatic movement of the eyes towards it – this is clearly neither desirable nor the case. The direct connections between the superficial and deeper layers of the superior colliculus ensure that eye movements desired by the brain are generated very rapidly. The system involves a minimal delay between something new appearing, the decision of higher brain centres to look at it in more detail and its fixation by the eyes.

We have already seen how seeing and hearing interact in the brain to produce perceptions. They are also closely associated with the initiation of actions that redirect our senses to what should be attended to next. We have seen that eye movements are strongly

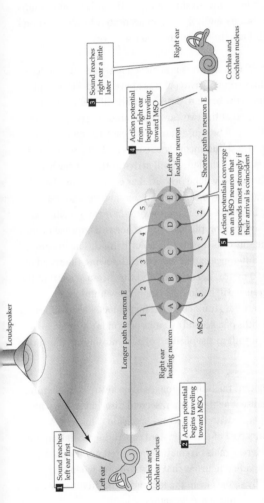

15. **Sound localisation by coincidence detection.** This diagram illustrates how neurons (from A to E) in a part of the brain called the medial superior olive (MSO) compute the location of a sound by the difference in the time of arrival of a sound at the left and right ears. In the example illustrated the sound source is closest to the left ear. The most sensitive neuron to a sound at this location will be neuron E. This is because the longer path to E from the left compensates for the delayed activation of the right ear. Action potentials therefore converge on neuron E at the same time (coincidence) and this double excitation of E will signal to the brain the location of the sound. Other neurons, when activated by coincident input from the left and right, signal other locations

influenced by novel objects appearing in the peripheral visual field. They are also affected by sound; we tend to want to look at what we are listening to. Our ability to shift our gaze towards a sound source depends on the brain's auditory system accurately localizing sound by integrating information from the two ears.

An important way in which this is achieved for sound frequencies below about 1 kHz (roughly two octaves above middle C on a piano keyboard) requires the brain to detect minute differences in the arrival time of sound at the two ears. If a sound source is directly ahead or behind it will be equidistant from each ear and sound will therefore arrive simultaneously at each ear. If the sound is directly to one side, say the left, it will arrive at the left ear before the right and the sound will be perceived as coming from the side of the leading ear. The interaural time difference for a sound arising directly from one side is the maximum it can possibly be since in any other position the time difference will approach zero – as it is when the source is directly ahead or behind. The maximum interaural time difference can be calculated knowing the speed of sound in air (340 metres per second) and the distance apart of the ears. This difference will be no more than a few hundred millionths of a second. Humans can in fact detect a time difference of just 10 millionths of a second (10 microseconds), a time associated with a shift in the position of a sound source by just one degree.

It is astonishing that the brain manages to be aware of such minute differences because it achieves microsecond discrimination using neurons that operate with millisecond precision. This feat is accomplished in a part of the brainstem called the medial superior olive or MSO. Here signals originating in the left and right ears converge on individual neurons that only respond when excited simultaneously by signals from the left and right. In other words these neurons are coincidence detectors.

The system computes difference in the time of arrival of a sound in the two ears because different coincidence-detecting neurons are sensitive to different interaural time delays. To do this neurons are organized anatomically such that signals resulting from a sound arriving at the left ear say 100 microseconds before arriving at the right are sent along neural pathways that differ in length. The path length differences introduce different delays and these are arranged so that signals initially separated in time converge simultaneously at a coincidence-detecting neuron. That neuron will be excited by the coincidence of its excitatory input and its firing will therefore represent an interaural time of 100 microseconds, the left ear leading. The brain will therefore interpret the firing of that neuron as a sound from the left. Many coincidence detectors in the left and right MSOs compute for the brain the location in space of relatively low frequency sounds.

For frequencies above about 2 kHz, computing the source of a sound is rather more straightforward because for higher frequencies the head casts a significant acoustic shadow. Sound coming from the left therefore seems louder in the left ear than the right. So the brain is furnished with information about the location of a sound source by two different neural computations, one depending on interaural time difference and the other on interaural sound intensity. The pathways mediating these two converge in the midbrain, providing the perceived location of a sound source, information required by the brain to redirect your attention should it choose to.

Internal senses also control actions

Our actions are strongly influenced by sensations originating in the body, of which we are generally not conscious. These senses are important because they inform the brain about the position of our limbs, muscle force and length, blood pressure, body temperature, our hunger and thirst, and so on.

That we are consciously aware of only a small fraction of the many sensations upon which our smoothly and efficiently executed actions depend can be illustrated by the following. Imagine thirst initiates a decision to drink a glass of water. You locate an empty glass, hold it under a tap and turn on the flow of water. We do not question our ability to hold the glass in a fixed position, in spite of the obvious fact that it becomes substantially heavier as it fills. How do we do that? Adopting an inelegant solution, you might generate lots of tension in antagonistic muscles of the arm and lock the elbow joint in position. More intelligently, you could watch the water flowing into the glass and deliberately increase the firing rate of motor neurons to adjust the muscular force required to compensate for the increasing weight of the glass. In this way you never have to exert any more energy than is necessary to hold the glass in place. This solution to the task would require you consciously to monitor the water's flow rate visually and then, according to one's experience of such things, anticipate the rate of increase in muscular force required to allow for the computed increase in the weight of the glass.

The visual cortex may well have enough computing power to solve the glass-filling problem easily, but the brain actually delegates the problem to a much lower level in the nervous system. In this way we do not need to be consciously aware of the trivial computations involved in the simple act of obtaining a glass of water. You can quench your thirst thoughtlessly by relying on a sense that never enters consciousness, namely the ability to monitor the length of skeletal muscles. Special sensory structures called muscle spindles are incorporated into the fabric of our skeletal muscles and monitor the length of the muscle, information that enables muscles to compensate automatically for increasing loads.

To see how this works we'll consider the biceps and triceps, antagonistic muscles affecting the elbow joint. As the weight of the glass increases, the biceps will lengthen a little, exciting sensory neurons in the muscle spindles causing them to fire nerve impulses at a higher frequency. This information about the change in length is transmitted into the spinal cord by sensory axons, which form excitatory synapses with motor neurons that innervate the biceps. Consequently the biceps generate more force, compensating for the increasing load. The sensitivity of the muscle spindles is so high that the desired length of the biceps muscle is restored quickly and the position of the hand is maintained, even in the face of a rapidly increasing load. In addition to exciting flexor motor neurons, the spindle sensory neurons of the biceps also excite inhibitory inter-neurons in the spinal cord. These reduce the activity of the motor neurons innervating the antagonistic triceps muscle. So at the same time that the biceps is producing more force, the triceps muscle generates less.

The reflex that responds to muscle stretch is one of many incredibly useful automatic control systems operating at the level of the spinal cord. Spinal cord neural circuits underlying these reflexes enable the brain to initiate complex intentional movements without having to bother to specify precisely how the motor neurons must act. The spinal cord also contains useful non-reflexive neural circuits relieving the brain of the responsibility for co-ordinating movements of the body and limbs during locomotion. Complex repeated patterns of motor neuron activity co-ordinating the contractions of many muscles are involved, for example, in the simple act of walking. Once again we see that the brain does not have a role in orchestrating the detail of the rhythmic pattern of neural activity required for walking or running. Neural circuits in the spinal cord, called central pattern generators, produce the appropriate basic patterns of motor activity for each gait. Sensory feedback from muscle and joint receptors fine-tunes the basic pattern, reinforcing it and making adjustments for variations in terrain.

Chapter 6
Memories are made of this

Our ability to modify our behaviour in response to life's experiences is shared by all animals and is a reflection of the brain's willingness to learn. Learning results in the formation of memories and in humans this process reaches its most sophisticated form, allowing us creatively to associate different reflections on the past, to generate new ideas, and most importantly to acquire language as a medium of expression and communication. Memory requires the brain to be physically altered by experience and it is this remarkable property that makes thought, consciousness, and language possible. So what do we know about memory, its nature, precise locations in the brain, and causes? Exactly what is altered in the brain when we learn and remember something?

Types of memory

We can all recognize that there are many different kinds of memory. The most basic distinction is between short-term and long-term memory. When you think about it, most of our memories must be fleeting because few of the many experiences we have in the course of an average day are remembered for very long, nor do they need to be. This should not be regarded as a failing or impairment of the brain's memory systems. On the contrary, transient memories are absolutely essential to the process of understanding the meaning of events as they occur in the present. This type of very short-term memory for things being experienced now is known as working memory; it allows you to comprehend what you are reading or to figure out the meaning of what has just been said to you in a conversation. Working memory can be thought of as a low capacity information reservoir that is always full, sensations flowing into it continuously at about the same rate that they are forgotten. A memory need only be in the reservoir just long enough to allow you to comprehend what's going on in the present. From this perspective you can see that forgetting, far from being a problem, is for many everyday purposes an absolutely essential and active element of the process of interacting effectively with a changing environment. Working memory is an indispensable form of transient memory; it a moving window of comprehension that allows us to understand the present in terms of the very recent past.

Importantly, working memory has a crucial role in comprehending spoken and written language. It allows you to keep track of meaning in the flow of words, as they are being heard or read. This close association between this form of memory and language is reinforced by brain imaging studies indicating that language-associated working memory is located in the frontal and parietal lobes of the cerebral cortex on the same side of the brain required for speech (left).

Some of the information held in short-term storage may be important enough to be remembered for a long time and must therefore be transferred to a more stable form of storage. Neuroscientists and psychologists trying to understand how long-term memories are formed have found that memories do not necessarily take a gradual path along which the probability of forgetting becomes progressively less and less likely. Rather it appears that learning activates a discontinuous process involving two distinct phases and physical mechanisms. It seems that short-term memories, such as memory for a telephone number just given to you, have an intrinsically unstable physical representation in the brain. Memories that are selected for consolidation become incorporated into a more-or-less permanent store, which must be represented by far more robust alterations in the brain's chemical and physical make-up.

Many factors contribute to determining whether particular short-term memories are transferred into the long-term store or are simply forgotten. Surprisingly our experiences do not necessarily have to be important to be remembered for a long time. For example, we are all familiar with the phenomenon of the 'flash bulb memory', the vivid memory we have of precisely what we were doing when for instance we first saw the news of the 9/11 attack on the World Trade Center. Of course we remember the important details of that grave event, but we also remember many trivial facts associated with what we were doing at the time. These are memories that in normal circumstances would certainly have been quickly forgotten. Flash bulb memory shows that emotional association is a powerful facilitator of long-term memory formation. There are other facilitators of permanent memory formation, most of which unfortunately require more deliberate action on our part, such as dogged practice and rehearsal.

The distinction between short-term and long-term memory provides a focus for thinking about how the brain is altered by the formation of a memory. We must assume that both types of memory require that something physical in the brain, its chemical and/or electrical properties, must be altered. For short-term memories the changes are transient whereas the changes associated with long-term memories must be permanent. Therefore they would seem to require different mechanisms for their formation and experimental work on animals supports this conclusion. Animal experimentation also shows that memory formation involves alteration or modulation of the properties of synapses in neural circuits. It may also require the formation of new synapses and changes in the electrical excitability of neurons. As for the distinction between short- and long-term memory formation, experiments show that in all cases the most important underlying distinction between the mechanisms is that the latter requires a dialogue between synapses and genes and the former does not. I will return to the physical mechanisms of permanent memory formation, but first it is worth considering the different kinds of long-term memory from a psychological perspective.

Life would be difficult without the ability reliably to store and to recall lots of commonplace facts, the names of our friends and acquaintances, telephone numbers, our way home after school or work, etc. These are explicit or semantic memories and they constitute our declarative knowledge. We know that neurons are nerve cells, that Edinburgh is the capital city of Scotland, that water will turn to ice at zero degrees, and that you must first boil water to make a cup of tea. Declarative knowledge is essential to the understanding of how things work and thus to an understanding of the world we live in. It is a body of knowledge that helps us to regulate our behaviour according to and dependent on reliable factual memories. Navigational skills, for example, depend on our ability to deploy a complex store of declarative knowledge, including detailed spatial memories and representations of the world. We assume all of the facts that constitute our knowledge of things must be stored in an organized fashion to be useful. Though this has not been demonstrated, it seems likely that the brain stores our semantic memories as modules that have some logical links to one another; they are grouped by category for instance. When we are trying to recall some fact, for instance the name of an acquaintance, our brain knows where to find the memory because it belongs to a particular category that is stored in a particular location or has a particular address in the brain.

Our brain's memory banks, however, do much more for us than store lots of useful facts. One important non-factual category of memory is procedural knowledge. This is the consequence of learning how to do something difficult such as riding a bicycle, knitting, or tying one's shoelaces. These are certainly difficult skills to acquire, but once learnt they are never forgotten, even without occasional practice. Thus it seems that the knowledge or information required for the execution of very complex motor routines or procedures is somehow laid down in a robust permanent memory store. The parts of the brain involved in the acquisition of complex motor skills are the basal ganglia and the cerebellum. Motor skills are an essential part of our memory store, but it is difficult to describe the 'know-how' in words. In this sense the memory is said to be implicit; you cannot explain how to ride a bicycle, whereas you could explain quite effectively your explicit memory for how to make a cup of tea.

Episodic memory corresponds to our memories of past events or episodes. Notice that our memory for episodes differs in important respects from our remembering of facts. First, we can acquire a memory for a fact gradually – learning a new telephone number for example may require several attempts. But a remembered episode, a childhood visit to the zoo, is a memory for a unique event that only happened once and there is no opportunity for learning the event by rehearsal. Secondly, a fact is a fact, our semantic memory for a new telephone number is therefore either true or false. The memory can easily be verified and two people's true memory for the same number will of course be the same. Episodic memories are not so easily verified. My sister and I may have very different memories of that visit to the zoo. So episodic memories are personal, highly selective, idiosyncratic, and possibly false, but they may also be richly complex and movie-like in character. They constitute the stories we tell ourselves about our past, they are the things we would write about in our autobiography. Episodic memories can be recalled deliberately or are triggered by evocative sensory stimuli. A particularly powerful stimulus evocative of episodic memory is the sense of smell. Exactly why this should be so is unclear, as the sense of smell is not well developed in humans and it links with primitive brain centres in the hypothalamus (see Chapter 5).

Because you can be surprised by an evoked memory of an episode you were not aware you had, there is uncertainty about exactly how much of our past is stored but not generally available to us. The evocation of vivid recollections that you were unaware had been memorized suggests that not everything is accessible by deliberate attempts at recall. Evidence for this was first provided in the 1940s by the American neurosurgeon Wilder Penfield (1891–1976). Penfield studied medicine at Oxford where in 1914 he was inspired by the influential British neurophysiologists Charles Sherrrington (1852–1957), the scientist who coined the terms neuron and synapse and whose work on many aspects of the mammalian nervous system won him the Nobel Prize in 1932. In 1934 Penfield founded the Montreal Institute of Neurology and there performed many operations on conscious epileptic patients during which he electrically stimulated small regions of the cerebral cortex. In the course of the operations patients reported very detailed memories of long past events. When he stimulated the same small area again the same memory popped into the patient's mind, memories about things or events that otherwise were not recalled.

These experiments did show that episodic memories may not be readily recallable, but some have wrongly interpreted these experiments to mean that *every* past episode is stored. Most importantly, however, Penfield had found the first evidence for a physical basis of memory. The fact that the same memory was evoked by repeated stimulation in the same place suggested that specific memories not only have a physical basis but that each also has a particular physical location in the brain.

The 'where' of memory

As we have seen, various labels are used to describe different types or categories of memories. The categories are not just a convenient classification system of academic interest only. Explicit working memory for example is associated with the pre-frontal cortex. The hippocampus is likely to be the part of the brain where working memories are transferred into long-term explicit memories.

Damage to the hippocampus prevents the formation of new declarative memories, but does not affect the brain's ability to learn new procedural skills. The hippocampus is also implicated in stores of spatial memories required for effective navigation. In rats and mice it contains neurons known as place cells that fire bursts of action potentials when the animal is in a particular place. When synaptic transmission in the hippocampus is disrupted animals are unable to learn to navigate around mazes. Structural brain scanning (MRI) in humans indicates that the hippocampus stores detailed mental maps that help us to navigate. Interestingly, as more spatial information is stored in the human hippocampus the structure becomes larger. Thus London taxi drivers, who store huge amounts of spatial information, have significantly larger hippocampi than people who do not drive taxis and moreover this is the only brain region that is affected. For procedural or motor memory it seems that the hippocampus is not required. Learning complex motor tasks engages the motor and sensory cortex, the basal ganglia, and the cerebellum. So different types of memories are acquired and stored by different brain regions.

Contributing to this body of understanding of where things happen are imaging techniques such as fMRI and PET that can identify the parts of the brain that are active while simple tasks are being performed and learned. While it is of course important to know *where* learning and memory happen, a far more important and fundamental question is *how* our memories are stored, that is to say, what is the biological nature of a memory's physical representation in the brain?

The 'how' of memory

It is difficult if not impossible to directly study the physical mechanisms of memory formation and storage in the human brain. Does this mean that we will never understand the physical basis of human memory? Probably not, because insights into the physical basis of human memory formation can almost certainly be achieved

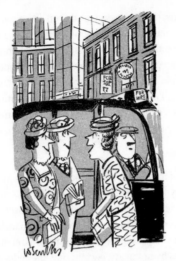

"We're in luck! He knows of a back-street cinema showing a 'U' film."

16. Taxi driver

through the study of brains far simpler than our own. We have already seen how our current understanding of electrical signalling in the human brain depended on experiments performed on a giant axon in the squid, a mollusc. In the field of learning and memory we will see shortly that another mollusc, a sea slug, has provided an almost ideal model system in which to study the most fundamental mechanisms of memory formation in the brain.

There are many other examples of this kind of thing in modern biology. For instance, practically everything we know about inheritance, DNA, and the genetic code is based on experiments performed on such unlikely and lowly subjects as the sweet pea, the fruit fly *Drosophila*, and a few species of bacteria and virus. This reductionism strategy works so effectively because biological systems are so remarkably conservative. So much so that my genes and yours use the same genetic code as worms, flies, chrysanthemums, brewers' yeast, and even slime mould for that matter, and our neurons use the same electrical and chemical signalling mechanisms as in the most humble of animals. The reductionist strategy in modern biology has been spectacularly successful in explaining the complex while investigating the relatively simple. Perhaps then amongst Nature's more modest animals there is a simple instance of learning and memory that would illuminate the secrets of the physical basis of our own memories?

The challenge of finding an ideal model animal in which a physical basis of memory formation might be revealed was one taken up in the 1960s by Eric R. Kandel, who trained as a psychiatrist and had started his studies of learning and memory in mammals. When Kandel embarked on his quest for a simple model of memory formation it was by no means certain that the reductionist approach would shed any light at all on something as sophisticated as memory in higher animals including man. In the year 2000 Eric was awarded the Nobel Prize in Physiology or Medicine for his universally important discoveries of how memories are formed in an animal incalculably simpler than man.

Kandel's search settled on a giant sea slug called *Aplysia californica*. The *Aplysia* brain has about 20,000 neurons, some of which are large enough to be visible to the naked eye. *Aplysia* can learn and most importantly the mechanisms and principles involved in its formation of short- and long-term memories are conserved throughout the animal kingdom, including in man. The behaviour Kandel and his co-workers selected for study is a protective reflex in which the sea slug withdraws its gill into the safety of the mantel cavity in response to a mild touch stimulus to another part of the body called the siphon. If the stimulus to the siphon is repeated a number of times, the gill withdrawal reflex becomes weaker until finally the animal ignores the touch stimulus. The waning of sensitivity to repeated stimulation is known as habituation and is a very simple form of learning found in all animals, including humans. It is clearly an adaptive behavioural mechanism as it prevents us from attending to stimuli which because of their repetition and evident lack of consequence can be of little or no danger, interest, or importance. The ticking of a grandfather clock in a small room for example may be quite loud, but we quickly habituate to it and the sound seems to fade.

Another type of learning, seen in humans and the sea slug, is sensitization. Sensitization occurs when we are exposed to an unexpected or strongly unpleasant stimulus. After such a stimulus our attention is alerted or sensitized and we are likely to become more responsive to what might previously have been regarded as innocuous stimuli. We can understand this in human terms if we again consider the ticking of the grandfather clock, a sound to which we had become habituated. Imagine that suddenly the clock chimed loudly, or that you experienced some other startling stimulus. Now our senses are heightened and we become instantly aware of the ticking clock again. Sensitization has quite abruptly reversed the effects of habituation. If nothing else untoward happens, we will soon become habituated to the clock and again 'learn' to ignore its ticking. Generally the sensitizing effect of a single alarming stimulus is short-lived, lasting perhaps for just a few minutes. In this case sensitization is a simple form of short-term memory. But if the alarming stimulus is repeated a number of times our senses may be heightened for days and now sensitization is a form of long-term memory.

So by using the simple paradigm of habituation and sensitization, Kandel has studied the two most basic types of memory, short-term and long-term. Most importantly he could observe precisely what was going on in individual neurons and at individual synapses while the memory was being formed. First Kandel showed that the gill withdrawal reflex of *Aplysia* can be sensitized by a single strong electric shock to the tail. Following the shock the defensive withdrawal of the gill in response to the weak siphon stimulus is much stronger. Thus a single shock gives rise to a memory in the

93

form of an enhanced or sensitized responsiveness, lasting just a few minutes. Next Kandel repeated the tail shock five times in spaced trials and converted the short-term memory into a long-term memory that lasted days. These elegant behavioural experiments dramatically demonstrated that *Aplysia* displays forms of learning leading to short- and long-term memory formation that are in essence strikingly similar to corresponding forms of learning in humans. What was required now was evidence that the similarity was deeper than mere resemblance; that there was indeed a true conservation of the physical or molecular mechanisms underlying memory formation between *Aplysia* and mammals.

In mammals it was well known that the biochemical requirements for short- and long-term memory formation were fundamentally different, the latter requiring the synthesis of new proteins. Precisely the same result was found in *Aplysia*, namely that long-term sensitization of the gill withdrawal reflex required new protein synthesis but short-term sensitization did not. This was the first unequivocal evidence that the basic molecular machinery underlying memory formation in *Aplysia* and mammals might be the same. In *Aplysia*, however, because its nervous system is relatively so simple, there was a realistic hope that the fundamental cellular and molecular mechanisms of memory could be directly determined for the first time.

The neuronal network controlling the gill reflex is simplicity itself. The sensory neurons that innervate the siphon, and which respond to touch, synapse directly on the motor neurons, excite them, and cause the gill to be withdrawn. On first inspection this neural circuit would seem to be too invariant and insufficiently complex to allow learning to occur. There is however another class of neuron associated with the circuit that acts precisely where the sensory neurons synapse with the gill motor neurons. The sensitizing stimulus to the tail excites these neurons and when they are inhibited the sensitizing effects of stimulating the tail are blocked. The activation of these neurons is therefore necessary for the sensitization memory to be formed. These key cells are called 'modulatory neurons' because, while they do not participate directly in the generation of the behaviour, they modulate (alter) the size and duration of the behavioural response. In the absence of activity in the modulatory neurons the sea slug is perfectly capable of performing the defensive gill withdrawal, but the strength of the response to touching the siphon is not capable of being enhanced in the short or long term by shocks to the tail.

Understanding the role of the modulatory neurons therefore became the crucial task in explaining how the strength of the gill reflex was modified by experience. This is precisely what Kandel and his co-workers were able to do. Their experiments showed that the activation of the modulatory neuron strengthened the pre-existing synapses between the sensory neurons and the motor neurons. Touching the siphon now produced an enhanced reflexive response. Moreover they showed that the neurotransmitter of the modulating neuron is serotonin (also known as 5HT) and that when a single puff of serotonin is directed at the sensory to motor neuron synapse, the synapse was strengthened for a few minutes – just as it is when the tail is stimulated with a single shock. If four or five puffs of serotonin are delivered in succession, the result is a long-term strengthening of the synapse. Thus serotonin alone can substitute for tail shock, producing either short or long-term synaptic memory depending on whether a single puff or five spaced puffs are delivered to the synapse. So now the questions about memory formation were reduced to understanding precisely how serotonin, a neurotransmitter found in all animals including man, strengthens a synaptic connection in both the short and long term.

Kandel showed that the common denominator explaining both short- and long-term memory in *Aplysia* is the ubiquitous second messenger called cyclic-AMP (see Chapter 3), whose synthesis in the sensory neurons is triggered by the action of serotonin released from the modulatory neurons. When cyclic-AMP is injected into the sensory neurons it mimics the effects of the puffs of serotonin.

Now we must ask how cyclic-AMP operates in the sensory neuron and how it causes short-term memory in response to a single puff of serotonin and long-term memory after a few puffs. This is quite complicated but the basic idea is that cyclic-AMP activates an important type of enzyme called a kinase, which modifies the properties of particular target proteins by adding a phosphate molecule to them; the term for this is protein phosphorylation. The target for this modification in the sensory neuron is a potassium channel protein. You may recall that a potassium channel is important in the downward phase of the nerve impulse (see Chapter 3). Importantly, in the sensory neuron the phosphorylated form of this channel behaves more slowly and this sluggishness delays the restoration of the sensory neuron's resting potential. The net result of this is a prolongation of the action potential in the sensory neuron and so more neurotransmitter is released by the sensory neuron. Thus the sensory neuron's synapse with the gill motor neuron is strengthened.

Finally, we have arrived – after a complex chain of events, initiated by tail-shock, we have strengthened a synapse and modified the animal's behaviour in the short term. This is only a short-term memory because special enzymes quickly remove phosphates from proteins and return them to their original state, restoring the synaptic strength to its lower pre-sensitized level. Notice that for the formation of a short-term memory there is a requirement for protein modification locally at the synapse, but there is no requirement for new proteins to be synthesized. This was expected because it had been known for some time that short-term memories are formed even when all protein synthesis is prevented. Blocking the synthesis of new proteins, however, prevents long-term memory formation and this is as true in *Aplysia* as it is in us.

Protein synthesis is initiated following the activation of a gene and the genes reside in the nucleus of the cell body, which for a neuron can be a long way from the synapses. Now Kandel had to explain how a long-term strengthening of a synapse, that requires the involvement of the nucleus, could be achieved by the repetitive application of serotonin to the synapse and not to the cell body. The inescapable conclusion was that local events at the synapse must somehow initiate a dialogue with the remote cell body and its nucleus. The conversation between synapse and nucleus results in the activation of the genetic information needed for the synthesis of the new protein required by the synapse for strengthening it in the long term. The initial steps in the process must be the same as were required for short-term memory because serotonin-stimulated cyclic-AMP synthesis results in both short- and long-term memory formation, depending on whether the serotonin is delivered just once or a few times in succession. Following repeated serotonin delivery, the level of cAMP-activated kinase is much higher and this allows the crucial step in the formation of long-term memory to occur. This crucial step is the transport from the synapse to the cell body of kinase molecules that have been activated by cyclic-AMP.

Once in the cell body the activated kinases enter the nucleus and there, in cooperation with other similar molecules, they modify special proteins that interact directly with DNA and thereby regulate the expression of particular genes. Through this mechanism some genes are turned on immediately (called immediate early genes) and others are turned on later. In *Aplysia* proteins that result from this process of gene activation are transported back to the synapse where they are used to maintain the strength of synapses already affected by local effects of cyclic-AMP and to grow new synaptic connections. So in *Aplysia* the conversion of a short-term into a long-term memory involves the reinforcement of the short-term changes in synaptic strength and the growth of new synapses, both of which require the synthesis of new proteins.

Memory mechanisms are universal

What lessons have we learnt from the many elegant experiments performed on the behaviour and relatively simple brain of the sea slug? For me two fundamental sets of conclusions stand out. First, we have seen that a crucial target of adaptive change in the brain of any animal is the synapse. Synaptic change or plasticity is fundamental to learning and memory formation. The chemical synapse has built-in molecular machinery whose only function is to alter the strength of that synapse. It also embodies the ability to communicate with the cell's genome, with the express purpose of effecting further change or consolidating short-term changes made locally at the synapse. The synapse is capable of initiating a dialogue with the genes that results in new proteins being transported back to the synapse, all in the interests of synaptic plasticity. Seen from this perspective, the synapse is a highly responsive, dynamic, and active participant in the essential process of responding to the changing environment. Neurons are not joined together with the biological equivalent of solder joints in an electronic circuit. The joints are not fixed but fluctuate in strength in accordance with experience. In this way behaviour is adapted continuously according to the latest experiences in our ever-changing surroundings.

Secondly, we have seen that built into the very structure of the genome are molecular mechanisms that allow experiences to change the pattern of gene expression in the brain. This is an example of how the distinction between nature and nurture is a particularly unhelpful way of thinking about how the brain works. One hears the question asked: are our mental abilities determined by our genes or our environment – by our nature or our nurture? Yet within the very nature of the brain is the machinery that allows it to respond adaptively to nurture. Our ability to learn from experience, to benefit from nurture, is allowed by the way our genes are designed to respond to experience.

I have described in some detail experiments performed on the lowly sea slug. Fascinating though these may be, do they throw light on how memories are formed in a brain as complex as our own? Is a dialogue between synapses and genes, for example, involved in the formation of the complicated types of explicit and implicit human memories already discussed? Indeed is it even possible that the same types of neurotransmitters, receptors, second messengers, and even the same genes are as important to human memory formation as in the sea slug?

The short answer to these questions is yes, and it is unlikely that Eric Kandel would have been awarded the Nobel Prize for his work had this not been the case. Of course there are differences in the details but, at the level of cells, molecules, and genes, the mechanisms of memory formation in slugs and human beings are remarkably similar, if not identical. Let us for example return to the mammalian brain and in particular to the hippocampus, a structure that in people with particularly good spatial memories (such as London taxi drivers) grows physically larger. The mammalian hippocampus is involved in explicit spatial memory and in the consolidation of short-term memories into a longer term storage. Although for spatial memory it is not clear precisely how information is stored in the hippocampus, it is well established in the mouse and rat brain that certain synaptic connections in the hippocampus are strengthened following bursts of stimuli applied to pre-synaptic neurons. Thus in the hippocampus there are synapses whose strength can be strengthened by activity. Just as in *Aplysia*, a single burst of activity results in short-term synaptic strengthening which does not require new proteins to be synthesized whereas repeated trains of stimuli results in a long-lasting strengthening that does require protein synthesis.

The similarities of the mechanisms of synaptic strengthening in the snail and the mammal are remarkable. Both have protein synthesis independent and dependent phases, corresponding to short- and long-term effects on synaptic strength. Both involve the activation of kinases and the phosphorylation of synaptic proteins. In both cases the consolidation of the long-term effects on synaptic transmission requires a similar molecular signal from the synapse to enter the nucleus, to activate other proteins that regulate the expression of specific genes. Finally, in both cases the new proteins synthesized as a consequence of the altered gene expression results in stabilizing the strength of existing synapses and in the formation of new synapses.

Our understanding of what memories are made of at the level of cellular and molecular mechanisms is quite sophisticated. It is advanced enough that we can reasonably expect it to lead to the development of 'smart' drugs to improve our ability to learn and perhaps even to aid in the recall of established memories. Such drugs might, for example, enhance the effectiveness of neurotransmitters involved in activation of genes required for long-term memory formation. But we should be cautious. Of the higher levels of organization of memory we are largely ignorant. Thus we know little about how memories are selected for long-term storage, how different memories are categorized, or indeed how the brain makes memories available for easy recall. There are drugs that marginally enhance memory performance, most of which are related to nicotine, the addictive ingredient of tobacco. These and other drugs may provide some level of cognitive enhancement to the elderly suffering memory loss, but more significant drug-based benefits will depend on a far better understanding of the fundamental mechanisms of memory formation, recall, and forgetting than we currently have.

So the best advice to anyone seeking a better memory and recall ability is to continue to learn. As we have seen, the brain is an extraordinarily plastic and responsive machine. When laying down new memories it makes new proteins and forms new synapses; some regions of the brain literally grow in response to the information storage demands placed on them. But just as we grow older we lose muscle power so we lose brain power, in part because neurons die as we age and cannot be replaced. However, physical exercise can dramatically improve the physical condition of young and old alike and today's neuroscience is telling us that mental exercise can have an equally dramatic effect on the well-being of our plastic brains. The take-home message would seem to be 'use it or lose it'.

Chapter 7
Broken brain:
invention and intervention

One of the most exciting and potentially beneficial areas of brain research exists at the interface between neuroscience and the physical sciences of engineering, information technology, and robotics. Here biological and physical science converge in a new creative alliance that aims to exploit similarities and differences between the ways brains and computers work. The potential benefits of this research are as diverse as they are important. They include the possibility of creating brain–machine hybrids that will restore the brain's sensory and motor functions damaged by disease or accident. These devices may also expand the capabilities of the normal brain, making the bionic man of science fiction a reality. In addition, the synergy between neuroscience and computer science is capable of delivering a new generation of artificially intelligent agents, autonomous mobile robots, for example, to perform jobs we would prefer not to do ourselves. In this new interdisciplinary research area there are scientific and medical opportunities in two different directions. On the one hand computer science can be used to help us understand and control the workings of the brain. At the same time, knowledge of how the brain works might help us design better computers.

Computer scientists' interest in the neurosciences is quite understandable. After all, some aspects of what the brain does can be thought of as 'computational' and the digital computer is a compelling metaphor for the brain. But we must be careful not to see the brain as being like a computer in the same way that the heart is like a pump. The heart is not just *like* a pump, it *is* a pump; the brain is *not* a computer; at least not yet. It is possible to know everything about how the heart works by understanding how it functions as a pump. We cannot speak of the brain in a similar way. If our model of how the brain works is dominated by reference to the way computers work, we will ultimately fail to understand the brain because the most interesting thing it does – 'thinking' – is fundamentally not a computational process.

So, while being in some respects similar to a computer, the brain is able to perform tasks that computers and robots are more-or-less completely hopeless at, but which engineers would dearly love to achieve artificially. Take for example the mundane task of vacuuming a child's bedroom. Surely the state-of-the-art artificial intelligence, pattern recognition software, and robotics that enabled NASA to put a roving explorer on the surface of Mars ought to be more than sufficient to allow a handy autonomous robotic vacuum cleaner to be built. But you cannot yet buy a robotic vacuum cleaner smart enough to be trusted in a child's bedroom. Robots do not think, and moreover we have no idea how to write a programme for thinking. It would not be possible to programme a robot to clean a child's bedroom because you could not write an algorithm for the mind of the occupant. You would need to formalize what, in a particular child's world-view, is junk and what is treasure, and this is simply not possible. To make the task seemingly even less attainable, the child's treasures are moving targets; today's treasure may turn into tomorrow's junk. In short, for this commonplace task you need to have a theory about the mind of the child who occupies the room. Otherwise you'll spend more time retrieving small but priceless objects from a vacuum bag full of fluff than you spent cleaning in the first place.

The limited capacity of silicon-based computational devices to imitate even simple natural intelligent behaviour has led many of us to consider how to make computers more organic. The hope is that more powerful artificial intelligence, more closely resembling the natural form, might be possible if artificial agents were to incorporate non-linear information-processing mechanisms that are characteristic of real brains. While it is easy to get carried away with the impressive performance capabilities of today's computers, even NASA did not trust its robotic Martian explorer to wander around on its own, guided only by the intelligence of its on-board computers. The intelligence behind this robot was human, some 64 million miles away, and operating a (very) remote joystick. NASA couldn't trust the robot to behave autonomously, not because its computers were too small but because no current computer of any size could substitute adequately for human intelligence. The world's most powerful supercomputer weighs a tonne, is the size of an average room, and consumes energy at more than a million times the rate of the human brain while at the same time being no match for it on any measure of creative intelligence.

Although we can expect the pace of progress in computational power to continue, true intelligence will not simply emerge. If computers continue to follow Moore's law – the density of components in a computer doubles every 18 months – they are inevitably set on a path to exceed the packing density of components in the human brain, possibly by the end of this decade. But even if Moore's law holds indefinitely, there is no evidence whatsoever that this alone will lead to the emergence of truly human-like intelligence from a machine. One reason seems to be that the relationship between complexity, performance, and the information required to build computers and brains is not at all comparable for the two kinds of machine. A fly brain contains about 100,000 neurons, requiring building instructions contained in about 20,000 genes. A human brain with ten million times more components can be constructed with instructions contained in just twice the number of genes (the human genome contains about 40,000 genes). Clearly the human brain is many orders of magnitude more complex than a fly brain, but more importantly the increased complexity is accompanied by a completely novel set of properties. The human brain is a creative thinking machine; the fly's most certainly is not.

No doubt we are building ever more complex and faster computers at an impressive rate. But even the most complex artificial brains do not approach the efficiency or capability of a fly's brain. A fly can after all fly through a bush at high speed using an on-board computer the size of a full stop. Try replacing its brain with a supercomputer strapped to the poor fly's back – squashed flies don't fly! Conventional computers are so inefficient and inherently unintelligent that it is not surprising that computer scientists are now turning their attention to neuroscience for inspiration in the creation of a new generation of efficient and adaptively intelligent machines.

There are two ways in which neuroscience can be harnessed to inform future developments in computer science and artificial intelligence. In the first, biological neural mechanisms are simulated in silicon devices. In the second, real neurons and real neuronal networks growing *in vitro* interact directly with silicon devices.

Our tendency to consider similarities between biological and man-made devices, a tradition adopted by Descartes (see Chapter 2), has already been the source of inspiration for important developments in computer science. Computer scientists have audaciously borrowed terms and concepts from neuroscience in the design of silicon devices called 'artificial neural networks' (ANNs). In ANNs, neuron-like entities or nodes are connected together in extensive networks where they integrate inputs until an output firing threshold is reached, behaving much in the same way as real neurons do in real neural networks. The artificial networks can be trained to recognize and respond to complex patterns of input, they can be configured to function as the artificial nervous systems of mobile robots, or they can be 'evolved' by the application of genetic algorithms in order to incorporate additional processes borrowed from brain science.

Clearly these devices represent an indirect attempt to incorporate an abstraction of the biological medium of the brain into an entirely artificial system. At best conventional ANNs simulate a highly simplified version of the brain's neuron-to-neuron communication system. As we have seen in Chapter 3, there is more to the brain's signalling system than can be attributed to the synaptic wiring diagram alone. Conventional ANNs do not however incorporate artificial versions of modulatory neurotransmission or non-synaptic communication. Attempts to simulate the brain's chemical communication system have resulted in a new generation of ANNs inspired by recent research showing that neurons can communicate non-synaptically by releasing diffusing gases such as nitric oxide (NO). NO is produced by special neurons and it diffuses away in all directions into a volume of the brain that may contain many other neurons and synapses affected by it. The crucial feature here, which is simulated in a 'GasNet' ANN, is that by employing a diffusing transmitter one neuron can affect another without actually being 'synaptically' connected or wired to it. So GasNets include connectivity or synaptic wiring like conventional ANNs, but they also simulate gaseous modulatory communication. By featuring this additional form of communication, GasNets have proved to be more adaptive than conventional networks that rely on the simulation of synaptic connectivity alone.

There are two ways in which the GasNets outperform more conventional artificial networks. First, for the same computational power they employ fewer neurons and have a simpler architecture than conventional artificial networks, making them more efficient. Secondly, and more importantly, they are significantly easier to create by the application of a genetic algorithm. To take one example, a genetic algorithm can be used to evolve artificial nervous systems for mobile autonomous robots. The advantage of this artificial evolutionary approach is that we do not have to employ

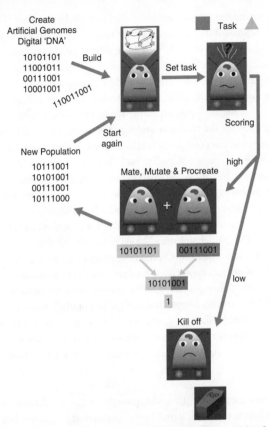

Create
Artificial Genomes
Digital 'DNA'

10101101
11001011
00111001
10001001
110011001

Build

Task

Set task

Scoring

high

Start
again

New Population

10111001
10101001
00111001
10111000

Mate, Mutate & Procreate

10101101   00111001

10101001

1

low

Kill off

17. **Artificial evolution of robot brain.** Artificial brains capable of solving 'real-world' problems that robots may encounter can be created by a process inspired by the evolution of real brains by natural selection. Each individual in a population of artificial neural networks is subjected to a fitness test, in this case to identify triangles and navigate towards them, avoiding squares. High scoring individuals 'mate' with one another, combining parts of their superior 'genetic' instructions. Mutations are also introduced in the creation of the next generation – a population of slightly superior individuals. These are subjected to the test again. After many hundreds of iterations of this cycle, a brain capable of guiding the robot reliably to triangles is created. This is achieved without requiring the robot scientists to design a brain for the task or even to understand how the evolved one works

conventional design engineering techniques in the creation of the robot's brain. All that is required is to specify the behavioural task you wish the robot to perform. The genetic algorithm generates a population (the first generation) of brains in which the neural circuits and mechanisms are specified by a computer code consisting of long strings of zeros and ones. These sequences can be regarded as digital DNA, providing the 'genetic' blueprint, instructions for the structure and function of the artificial brains. Each robot in the population is tested for its competence at the task and a fitness score is assigned to each. Initially of course, in the first generations, the fitness test enables one to say that one individual performs slightly less abysmally than another. This is followed by an explicitly elitist mating procedure in which the highest scoring individuals engage in simulated sex. Pairs of robots exchange parts of their 'DNA' which are recombined in the production of instructions for the brains of the next generation. At this stage mutations are incorporated at random into the instructions (consisting of changing a few zeros to ones and a few ones to zeros). This process results in an offspring population of slightly better or 'fitter' individuals, which are tested again, with a more stringent fitness criterion now being applied. At each test of fitness, poorly performing individuals in the population are killed off – so to speak.

The more complex the task, the more generations will need to be tested before the behavioural task is performed satisfactorily. But the number of generations is at least tenfold fewer if the genetic algorithm is evolving a GasNet rather than a conventional ANN. It seems therefore that by simulating diffusion and modulation in addition to synaptic connectivity, GasNets have the potential to out-perform more conventional ANNs. This is very encouraging because it suggests that if we go even further and incorporate even more realistic neural mechanisms into ANNs, we will improve our chances of creating more adaptive and perhaps more naturally intelligent artificial agents. Interestingly, in this evolutionary approach, computational devices wind up being nothing like those produced using the conventional wisdom of today's digital computer design.

Is it possible to imagine that thinking machines, perhaps even with consciousness, could be evolved using genetic algorithms? After all we have no idea how to design such a machine. So why try to understand the process when you can evolve it without necessarily being able to comprehend the relationship between the structure and its properties – which is reminiscent of our current level of understanding of how the real brain thinks.

In the second and even more audacious strategy, silicon chip technology is explicitly coupled with biology by growing a network of real neurons on the chip. In this way the silicon devices can communicate with the neurons and vice versa. Ultimately the aim is to construct, from living nerve cells interacting with an electronic medium, a super-intelligent computer with a human-like ability to think. Is it possible to imagine an organic computer of living neurons, a prosthesis for the brain, deriving its energy efficiently from oxygen and nutrients? We are a long way from this goal but a number of labs, including my own, are trying to grow neurons in such a way that they can be manipulated and interfaced with silicon devices – hybrids of carbon and silicon-based technologies. In this way, future computers may be able to harness the non-linear information-processing dynamics of neurons and thereby become truly intelligent.

The practical problems of this future technology present an enormous challenge and both approaches to more organic computing – the simulation and explicit interfacing of biological processes – are in their infancy. But the signs are positive. It is clear that biologically inspired computer technologies and computational methods offer the real prospect of a quantum leap in the ability of artificial systems to approach the levels of adaptive intelligence we take for granted in ourselves. This is not to suggest that advances in conventional computational technology have been slow-paced or merely incremental in character. Clearly this is not the case since processing speed, memory capacity, and miniaturization have advanced spectacularly over the past few decades. But arguably this pace ought to have brought us significantly closer to achieving machines that think for themselves than we currently are.

There seems to be no doubt that the influence of neuroscience on the next generation of computers will find all sorts of beneficial applications. Important among them will be medical technologies that depend on interfacing the brain with artificial electronic devices. Some of these are already effectively using conventional computer systems. But because these developments require computers to interact very directly with natural intelligence, this is an area that is likely to benefit enormously from the kind of biologically inspired organic computer technologies that we have considered and will emerge in the future.

Machines that fix the broken brain

There are two fundamentally different ways in which brains and artificial devices can be conjoined therapeutically. In the first, the implanted device electrically stimulates neurons to replace lost sensory function. In the second, an electronic device is placed on, in, or close to the brain and is used to detect electrical output signals from neurons. These signals are amplified and then processed in a computer so that they can control useful external electronic or mechanical devices. By potentially turning thoughts into action this technology holds the very real promise of restoring lost brain function, in particular with regard to re-establishing volitional control of movement. In both input (stimulating) and output (recording/detecting) types of brain–machine interface, the computer acts as a surrogate for the damaged brain. I will briefly consider both approaches and an application in which the stimulation of the brain is influenced by activity detected in the brain's output.

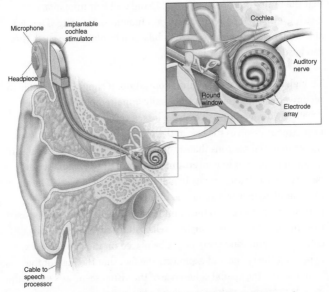

18. **Cochlear implant. Where the auditory hair cells that respond directly to sound are damaged or fail to develop, the sensory neurons they normally communicate with can be stimulated directly by a filamentous linear array of electrodes connected to a microphone and sound processor**

The most straightforward stimulating device used in humans is the cochlear implant. In most cases of hearing impairment the sound receptor hair cells are lost, but the sensory neurons that they excite and whose axons constitute the auditory nerve remain intact. With a cochlear implant, a small external microphone captures the sound waves and transforms them into electrical pulses. These are delivered, via multi-channel stimulating electrode arrays, to the sensory neurons in the cochlear. Generally the sound waves are digitized, so that they can be subjected to processing to enhance comprehension, especially of speech. The electrical stimulation of the neurons in the auditory nerve acts to transduce the artificially generated signal into trains of nerve impulses in the auditory nerve that the brain interprets as sound. Using cochlear implants, hearing-impaired patients can regain functional hearing. They are able to perceive speech and, when bilateral implants are used, they can localize sound (see Chapter 5).

Though a far more challenging proposition, it should be possible to restore at least partial sight to visually impaired people using a prosthetic device. As with hearing loss, a common cause of visual impairment involves the loss of the receptor cells in the retina rather than the neurons that transmit information to the brain. An artificial retina might convert images captured by a camera into patterns of electrical activity in a multiple electrode array. The array can stimulate neurons along the brain's visual pathway. If the pathway from the eye to the brain is intact, the implant can be used to stimulate the retinal ganglion cells. Alternatively a spatially coherent stimulating array might be placed on the visual cortex, bypassing the retina and exploiting the fact that the map of the visual world, the spatial coherence of the visual scene as seen by the eyes, is preserved and projected onto the visual cortex.

Brain–machine interfaces that involve the stimulation of neurons may also ameliorate some neurological disorders, such as Parkinson's disease and chronic pain. In Parkinson's disease, following the loss of neurons in the substantia nigra, the motor control functions of the basal ganglia nuclei are disrupted. These ganglia are involved in the activation of intentional movements and in this progressive disorder patients suffer from a frustrating inability to implement actions corresponding to their intentions. Stimulating electrodes implanted in the basal ganglia can fulfil some of the regulatory functions that have been lost, significantly improving the quality of life for Parkinson's sufferers.

It is in the combination of output and input brain–machine interface technology that particular promise for treatment of epilepsy is held. For some types of epileptic seizure, distinctive signals in the cortex precede the full epileptic attack, sometimes by minutes. A recording device might recognize these signals as the forerunners of an imminent seizure and that predictive information could be used to warn the patient or to activate a stimulating interface device to reduce the severity of the attack. The device might electrically stimulate neural pathways that reduce cortical epileptic activity or trigger an embedded drug delivery system. In this application of interface technology the patient has not one brain but two and the second, the computer, is designed to control the biological one, preventing it from doing something harmful to the patient.

With almost evangelical zeal, Miguel Nicolelis of Duke University in the USA has pioneered and promoted this type of technology, which he refers to as 'hybrid brain–machine interfaces' or HBMIs. He is very optimistic that in the future HBMIs will allow the brain to control computers and other artificial devices designed to replace brain functions lost through injury or disease. Nicolelis's initial experiments with primates, which provided proof of principle, were performed on a nocturnal owl monkey called Belle. By tapping into the activity of about 100 neurons in different regions of the monkey's cortex, he showed that different patterns of activity predicted and anticipated different specific reaching movements. The patterns representing intentions to carry out actions preceded the specific actions by a few fractions of a second.

More recently, using a macaque monkey, whose brain more closely resembles that of a human, Miguel Nicolelis has used patterns of neural activity recorded from the surface of the motor cortex to control the movements of a robot arm. In a remarkable demonstration of 'mind over machine' the macaque can learn, using visual feedback, to control the movements of a robotic arm, causing it to reach in particular directions in response to brain activity associated with similar movements of a joystick grasped by the monkey.

The monkey is rewarded with a sip of fruit juice for performing

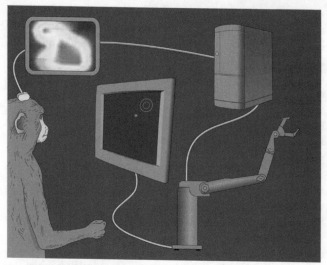

19. The monkey can be trained to use its thoughts to guide a robotic arm to reach for an object

joystick movements that guide a cursor to a target on the computer screen. The pattern of brain activity associated with that movement is used to drive a particular reaching movement of the robotic arm. Eventually the monkey realizes that it can receive the reward simply by thinking; by generating in its brain an intention to move the joystick. That intention is then translated computationally into a specific reaching movement of the robotic arm.

Obviously there are important medical applications of this research area. But beyond offering a beneficial therapeutic technique for the patient with a damaged brain, HBMIs could potentially lead to an unprecedented augmentation in normal brain performance, significantly extending the brain's power to interact with machines. This is a prospect both seductive and frightening and one that certainly demands serious ethical reflection. One area of application that deserves scrutiny is the military implications of HBMI technology, implications that have not escaped the attention of the US Defence Advanced Research Projects Agency, which is funding brain–machine interface research. Seriously provocative new weapons capabilities could be placed under the direct control of an individual's thoughts. This offers the edge over an adversary because time-consuming natural human reticence and ethical reflection would be neatly bypassed by coupling a thought directly to a firing trigger.

Notwithstanding these worries, HBMI technology has the potential to be enormously beneficial to patients in whom the connection between motor intentions originating in the cortex and the ability to move a limb has been broken by a spinal injury. In fact today's medical science can offer very little else because realistically we are probably decades away from being able to understand how to persuade the central nervous system to repair itself. Though there are developments that suggest regeneration therapies offer some hope, until such therapies are effective in restoring function to damaged pathways, brain–machine interface technology offers a realistic alternative and the bionic man is no longer necessarily the preserve of science fiction.

Of course the experiments on monkeys, showing that mind control of useful prosthetic devices is possible, involve highly invasive and expensive surgical procedures. In addition, with current technology a patient would be required to have his or her brain wired to some fairly cumbersome computer hardware to decode desired movement information from the brain to allow the patient to control the robotic device. We can anticipate that in the not too distant future wireless technologies and further miniaturization will enable a prosthetic limb to be controlled effortlessly by thought-intentions without the need for the patient to be tethered to a computer by unwieldy cables. But the implanting of microelectrode arrays on the appropriate regions of the cortex will still require major surgery.

This unavoidably invasive, and expensive, aspect of brain–machine interface technology has stimulated a renewed interest in non-invasive techniques using electroencephalography (EEG). Using electrodes placed on the scalp, EEG records electrical activity reflecting the summed actions of millions of neurons. There are doubts however whether such recordings will provide sufficiently high-resolution information of the brain's intentions. Notwithstanding the difficulties, advances are being made. Jonathan Wolpaw of the New York State Department of Health has shown that people with and without spinal cord injury can learn how to control their EEG patterns to move a cursor on a computer monitor. No doubt more needs to be done to make non-invasive interfacing work more effectively. But the necessarily very high cost and invasive character of brain–machine interfacing by electrode implantation will act as the mother of invention, and high-resolution non-invasive EEG methods coupled to more effective training and feedback paradigms ultimately will improve substantially.

There are other ways in which brain–machine interfacing might be made more patient-friendly and more effective in restoring lost motor function. One could dispense with the robotic prosthetic limb and arrange for the information about cortical intentions to be used to control the patients' own motor nerves or muscles. If the computer can transform cortical activity into an intention-associated pattern of electrical signals delivered to the actuators of a robotic limb, then it should also be able to deliver movement-specific signals to biological actuators – muscles. Direct control of motor nerves or muscles is obviously attractive, especially because injuries that result in paralysis generally do not damage the spinal motor circuits that are capable of controlling limb movements. It might be possible therefore to stimulate spinal motor circuits to produce co-ordinated limb movements without the need to target individual motor neurons. If successful, this technology will allow the patient to co-ordinate their movements with their own thoughts, in spite of the disconnection of the biological link between their brain and their spinal cord.

Can the broken brain fix itself?

A number of the applications of brain–machine interface technology are aimed at restoring motor or sensory function lost as a consequence of either injury or disease to the central nervous system. No matter how successful these techniques will become, it is likely that they will always be limited by the difficulty of artificially reproducing all of the functions performed by broken or damaged neuronal pathways. An alternative, and in many ways preferable, approach to restoring nervous system function will involve attempting to repair, rather than bypass, the affected neural pathway or region of the brain.

This represents a prodigious challenge. In contrast to peripheral sensory neural pathways, which can repair themselves and regenerate their original connections after injury, central neural pathways in the mammalian brain cannot. We do not know yet precisely why this distinction between peripheral and central nervous system repair capabilities should exist. Far more research is required to resolve the molecular and cellular mechanisms that determine whether damaged neurons can repair themselves or not, or whether dead ones can be replaced by new ones or not. This is an area of very active research, which we can only hope will shortly result in therapies to encourage broken neurons to regenerate lost connections and for dead neurons to be replaced.

Although the repair of spinal cord injury and the full restoration of function following spinal cord injury remain considerably beyond the scope of current medical science, fruitful lines of research have emerged and there is now good reason to be hopeful that in the not too distant future, spinal cord injury will be reversible. Much of the research effort is aimed at understanding why the central nervous system is unable to repair itself. Some experimental evidence points to the possibility that this is due to the presence of inhibitory molecular signals and to the absence of the type of growth-promoting molecules that are present in the periphery. In the adult brain, damaged myelin produces signals that prevent the regeneration of severed axons. In the developing brain however myelin supports the growth of young axons, and in the peripheral nervous system myelin contributes to the ability of peripheral axons to regrow following injury. It is as if in the adult central nervous system, but not in the young brain or in the peripheral nervous system, myelin produces substances that inhibit the regrowth of axons especially at the site of a lesion.

If these growth inhibitors could be neutralized, perhaps injured central axons would then regenerate and find their way to their targets again. The problem with this approach is that there are many growth-inhibiting molecules and only a few of them are known and characterized. Medicines that neutralize some of the molecules that inhibit growth have been developed, but they have a very marginal effect on regeneration. Unfortunately it appears that the effects of growth-inhibiting molecules are not simply cumulative – one or just a few of them are enough to prevent all regeneration. In an effective therapy therefore, most, if not all, of the myelin-derived inhibitors at the lesion site would have to be neutralized effectively to promote the regeneration of a damaged neural pathway.

Technical difficulties associated with the delivery of an effective and comprehensive neutralizer of all growth inhibitors has led some scientists to search for growth promoters to aid axon regeneration around, if not through, a site of injury in the brain. This approach, providing a growth-supportive bridge over the obstacles to regeneration, depends on exploiting the regeneration environment in which peripheral neurons live.

Another promising approach exploits an exception to the rule that neurons in the adult central nervous system do not grow and are not replaced. This exception is found in the mammalian olfactory system. Here new neurons continue to be produced throughout adult life. Once born, the new neurons extend an axon into the central nervous system to connect with the olfactory centres of the brain. Growing olfactory axons are sheathed by special myelin formed by the only glial cell type capable of crossing the boundary between the peripheral nervous system and the brain. These glial cells, called olfactory ensheathing cells, are unique in that they enable axons to fend off the inhibitory signals preventing the growth of other axons in the brain. In 1994 Ramon-Cueto and Nieto-Sampedro of the Ramon y Cajal Institute in Madrid showed that implanting these special cells allowed severed sensory axons to grow back into the spinal cord where they could reconnect with their targets and restore sensory function. Now many other scientists have shown that the regeneration-fostering properties of transplanted olfactory ensheathing cells may even be able to promote axonal growth across a severed spinal cord. Olfactory ensheathing cell transplantation is one of the most promising research strategies to improve treatment for spinal injury and offers a very real hope of an effective therapy.

Not broken, but not working properly

In some cases the brain is not physically broken by injury, stroke, or other insult, but nonetheless is still dysfunctional. With conditions such as depression, anxiety, amnesia, and schizophrenia it seems that the chemical communication systems of the brain, not its nerve pathways, are affected. Most common of all is depression, a debilitating condition that some 20–40 per cent of adults will experience at some time in their lives.

You will recall that there are two quite different types of chemical messengers or neurotransmitters in the brain. There are those that establish the brain's wiring diagram, ensuring either rapid excitatory or inhibitory connections between neurons in complex networks. These fast transmitters work by binding to special receptor molecules that directly activate the flow of electrically charged ions into or out of the affected neuron. It is thought that depression does not arise from a disruption to the brain's neural network. Rather it seems that the problem resides among the indirect neurotransmitters and it seems depression is a condition that reflects an abnormality of brain chemistry rather than brain structure. Strongly implicated in depressive disorders are the slow monoamine transmitters serotonin, noradrenalin, and dopamine. In the brain of a depressed person there is an insufficiency of these transmitters. Precisely how this causes the symptoms of depression, including loss of interest in life, lowered appetite, sleep disruption, and suicidal tendencies is not fully understood, though we do know that drugs that elevate the brain's monoamine levels can be an effective treatment for this illness.

This important class of drug is known as monoamine selective re-uptake inhibitors, a name that refers to their mode of action. In Chapter 3 we saw that, following the release of neurotransmitters, their action must be rapidly terminated so that a following chemical message is not confused with the previous one. The process of transmitter action termination is known as inactivation. Inactivation for serotonin and noradrenalin involves their removal from the region of the synapse by a selective re-uptake mechanism. By inhibiting a neurotransmitter's re-uptake it tends to accumulate in the brain, its concentration is increased, and over a period of weeks the depressive symptoms are reversed or ameliorated.

Antidepressants, the first of which were discovered more than 50 years ago, are now the most widely prescribed drugs. But depression remains the most prevalent of all psychological diseases and not all experts are convinced by the efficacy of commonly prescribed antidepressants, all of which increase the level of monoamine transmitters in the brain. In fact there is growing concern that the monoamine hypothesis is wrong and that some antidepressants may increase the likelihood of suicide. The fact is we know very little about the fundamental neurobiology of depression. It is very unlikely to be due simply to an insufficiency of monoamines. If this were the case, it would be difficult to understand why antidepressant drugs that raise monoamine levels quickly take several weeks to have a significant effect on depressive symptoms. This delay suggests that antidepressants work indirectly and that depression is caused by biochemical dysfunction that is only distantly linked to monoamine function. Indeed, in their search for new targets for antidepressant drugs, pharmaceutical companies are now exploring alternative biochemical pathways, such as those associated with the regulation of the brain's stress hormone cortisol. Growing concerns about the safety and side effects of the monoamine uptake inhibitors are a driving force behind the search for more effective new treatments for this baffling illness of the brain.

In this chapter we have seen how the broken brain might be fixed by a combination of brain–machine interface technology, the neutralization of inhibitors of regeneration, or by manipulating the nervous system's ability to repair itself. Brain dysfunction and injury is so frightening because it affects who we are, not just what we are. Effective treatments and cures are not yet available for many common disorders of brain function and perhaps this is not surprising: after all the brain is stupendously complicated. Nevertheless we can be encouraged by the pace of discovery in the neurosciences and optimistic that ultimately a better understanding of how the brain works will help us to fix it.

Chapter 8
Epilogue

Much can and has been learnt about the brain by determining where different mental tasks are performed and our ability to do so has been dramatically enhanced in recent years by the use of imaging technologies such as fMRI that allow the working brain to be functionally mapped. We should not however be seduced by beautiful pictures of the brain in action and there is the need for a mature evaluation of the contribution that localization of function by fMRI or other imaging technologies can make to an understanding of how the brain works as a whole.

It is important to recall that fMRI localizes neuronal activity indirectly by detecting changes in blood flow, and may therefore seriously misrepresent it. Certainly there is a link between increased blood flow and measures of neuronal activity, but the link may not be obligatory and at best it is likely to be decidedly rough. We know for instance that the brain can perform all of the functions required for recognizing a face within about 300 milliseconds, whereas it takes seconds for blood vessels to dilate. It is possible therefore that brief bouts of functionally important neural activity do not attract a blood surge. Also, where increased blood flow is detected in a region, it might be triggered by a number of quite different distinct bouts of neural activity involving different neurons performing different functional operations. The fMRI method is also unlikely to detect important functional operations that are not highly localized but performed by diffusely distributed networks of neurons. These may go undetected because the network functions without requiring more oxygenated blood. In other words there are likely to be important operations performed by neurons that can be achieved within the capacity of the normal blood supply to accommodate them. Actively working neurons may not need to whistle up more energy resources and so they will not be detected by fMRI.

Even if we grant that fMRI and other imaging technologies can produce reliable high-resolution maps of the brain's responses to different cognitive tasks, simply knowing where something happens is not the same thing as knowing *how* it happens. Our next challenge in neuroscience is to explain how the brain works as a whole, processing massive amounts of information in parallel. This is a challenge that will require us to leave behind a localizational way of thinking about the problem. We are left however with a paradoxical situation in which our most sophisticated understanding of the brain comes from highly local recordings of the electrical activity of one or just a few of its countless neurons at a time.

Will we ever understand completely how the brain works? If here the word 'understand' is used in the same sense that we can use it to indicate that we understand how a television works, I doubt it. Televisions are complicated and remarkable devices, but they were conceived by the human brain and built by the human hand. In spite of this, however, few of us would claim to have a complete understanding of how a TV works – sufficient to fix it when it doesn't for instance. Nonetheless, we trust that some knowledgeable individuals do know everything about televisions and the workings of televisions therefore leave no philosophical questions unresolved. Our understanding of how the brain works will probably not reach this level. Some future scientist may proclaim that he or she has attained a complete understanding of the brain. But it seems improbable that the rest of us would then simply stop regarding thinking, dreaming, poetry, and the beauty of a sunset as somewhat puzzling manifestations of the brain in action and the cause of some modest philosophical reflection.

Further reading

General Books

There are many excellent textbooks on the neurosciences but few that provide a comprehensive and accessible introduction for the non-specialist. However, both Fred Delcomyn's *Foundations of Neurobiology* (Freeman & Co., 1998) and *Essentials of Neural Science and Behaviour* by Eric R. Kandel, James H. Schwartz, and Thomas M. Jessell (Prentice Hall International, 1995) combine lucid text with unusually helpful illustrations and can be recommended for readers wishing to take the subject further. For a guide to the human mind see *Oxford Companion to the Mind*, 2nd edn., edited by Richard L Gregory (Oxford University Press, 2004).

Chapter 1

For a review of some of the most important literature on the control of eye movements in reading see Keith Rayner, 'Eye Movements in Reading and Information Processing: 20 Years of Research', *Psychological Bulletin*, 124 (1998), 372–422.

Chapter 2

The website *http://www.bri.ucla.edu/nha/histneur.htm* provides a number of useful links to authoritative resources on the history of neuroscience.

At *http://nobelprize.org/index.html* you will find information about the Nobel Prize awarded to Golgi and Cajal for their pioneering work discussed in this chapter. Also for a scholarly and comprehensive history of concepts about the brain in action see *Origins of Neuroscience: A History of Explorations into Brain Function*, by Stanley Finger (Oxford University Press, 2001).

Chapter 3

Both Fred Delcomyn's book *Foundations of Neurobiology* (Freeman & Co., 1998) and *Essentials of Neural Science and Behaviour*, by Eric R. Kandel, James H. Schwartz, and Thomas M. Jessell (Prentice Hall International, 1995) will be helpful in clarifying some of the difficult concepts touched on in this chapter. For a more technical but no less clear account see *An Introduction to Molecular Neurobiology*, by Zach W. Hall (Sinauer Associates, 1992).

Chapter 4

For a contemporary view on the animal evolution see Kenneth M. Halanych, 'The New View of Animal Phylogeny', *Annual Reviews of Ecology, Evolution and Systematics*, 35 (2004), 229–56. For more on the role of sexual selection in the rapid evolution of the human brain see *The Mating Mind: How Sexual Choice Shaped the Evolution of Human Nature*, by Geoffrey F. Miller (Doubleday, 2000).

Chapter 5

The website of Richard L. Gregory (editor of *Oxford Companion to the Mind* – see above), *http://www.richardgregory.org/index.htm*, is thought provoking on the elusive connection between sensation and perception, with some fascinating down-loadable illusion movies. For a contemporary reconsideration of the grandmother cell idea see R. Quian Quiroga *et al.*, 'Invariant Visual Representation by Single Neurons in the Human Brain', *Nature*, 435 (2005), 1102–7; Eric R. Kandel, 'The Molecular Biology of Memory Storage: A Dialogue between Genes and Synapses', *Science*, 294 (2001), 1030–8.

Chapter 6

For the original research article on the physical consequences of spatial learning in the brains of taxi drivers see Eleanor A. Maguire *et al.*, 'Navigation-Related Structural Change in the Hippocampi of Taxi Drivers', *Proceedings of the National Academy of Sciences*, 97 (2000), 4398–4403.

Chapter 7

For more on brain–machine interfaces see Miguel A. L. Nicolelis, 'Actions from Thoughts', *Nature*, 409 (2001), 403–7, and Aileen Constans, 'Mind over Machines', *The Scientists* (14 Feb. 2005), 27–9. For the latest on overcoming obstacles to regeneration in the adult mammalian spinal cord see Fouad K. Schnell *et al.*, 'Combining Schwann Cell Bridges and Olfactory-Ensheathing Glia Grafts with Chondroitinase Promotes Locomotor Recovery after Complete Transaction of the Spinal Cord', *Journal of Neuroscience*, 25 (2005), 1169–78.

Index

Index

Expand your collection of
VERY SHORT INTRODUCTIONS

Visit the
VERY SHORT
INTRODUCTIONS
Web site

www.oup.co.uk/vsi

➤ **Information** about all published titles

➤ News of **forthcoming books**

➤ **Extracts** from the books, including titles not yet published

➤ **Reviews** and views

➤ **Links** to other **web sites** and main OUP web page

➤ Information about **VSIs in translation**

➤ **Contact** the editors

➤ **Order** other **VSIs** on-line